NO LONGER PROPERT
THE SEATTLE PUBLIC L

D0020303

Praise for
Every Breath, New Chances

W8-BUA-783

"Make no mistake, this book is not just for men! *Every Breath, New Chances* is a wise and compassionate companion in the journey of aging. Lewis Richmond shares his own experiences of aging and provides Deep Mind Reflection exercises to explore inner feelings and other aspects of aging. He encourages the reader to meet these challenges as a rich opportunity for personal growth and development. For women, Richmond's insights are not only helpful for better understanding those in their life who are facing the fact that they no longer possess the virility, power, and control they once had, but also for understanding the feminine path of aging. This is a must-companion along the way."

—DIANE ESHIN RIZZETTO, author
of *Waking Up to What You Do*

"This is a book you can trust to guide you as you age! *Every Breath New Chances* is rooted in real wisdom and full of heart. It deepens many aspects of growing older and being a man without being too simple or too loud. Richmond really wants you to get more out of life. I'm about to turn eighty, and I feel better for having read it."

—THOMAS MOORE, author of
Care of the Soul

AUG 1 3 2021

"To process the mental and emotional challenges he faced growing older, Lewis Richmond says he wrote the book he needed. That sound writing advice has produced a one-of-a-kind toolkit with insights and practices that show others how to bring alive (and thus gain life-changing wisdom from) the book's profound core message: 'vulnerability is strength.'"

—PAULA SPENCER SCOTT, author
of *Surviving Alzheimer's*

"As my entire generation moves toward its end, I can't think of a more helpful, necessary book. Lewis Richmond offers a calm and systematic framework and practice to help you get the most out of your life right now! Why miss a second of it? Why not learn to love our growing old? This book will help you."

—PETER COYOTE, actor, writer,
Zen priest, and author of *Sleeping Where I Fall*

"*Every Breath, New Chances* is the first of its kind—an incredibly valuable book on male aging covering all the salient points. I highly recommend it, both for men and the women who care about them."

—LAMA PALDEN DROLMA, author
of *Love on Every Breath*

EVERY
BREATH,
NEW
CHANCES

Other books by Lewis Richmond

Work as a Spiritual Practice

Healing Lazarus

A Whole Life's Work

Aging as a Spiritual Practice

EVERY BREATH, NEW CHANCES

How to Age with Honor and Dignity

A GUIDE FOR MEN

LEWIS RICHMOND

Foreword by Peter Coyote

North Atlantic Books
Berkeley, California

Copyright © 2020 by Lewis Richmond. All rights reserved. No portion of this book, except for brief review, may be reproduced, stored in a retrieval system, or transmitted in any form or by any means—electronic, mechanical, photocopying, recording, or otherwise—without the written permission of the publisher. For information contact North Atlantic Books.

Published by
North Atlantic Books
Berkeley, California

Cover art by © gettyimages.com/GeorgePeters
Cover design by John Yates
Book design by Happenstance Type-O-Rama

Printed in the United States of America

Every Breath, New Chances: How to Age with Honor and Dignity is sponsored and published by the Society for the Study of Native Arts and Sciences (dba North Atlantic Books), an educational nonprofit based in Berkeley, California, that collaborates with partners to develop cross-cultural perspectives, nurture holistic views of art, science, the humanities, and healing, and seed personal and global transformation by publishing work on the relationship of body, spirit, and nature.

North Atlantic Books' publications are available through most bookstores. For further information, visit our website at www.northatlanticbooks.com or call 800-733-3000.

Library of Congress Cataloging-in-Publication Data

Names: Richmond, L. (Lewis), 1947- author.
Title: Every Breath, New Chances : How to Age with Honor and Dignity: A Guide
  for Men / Lewis Richmond.
Description: Berkeley : North Atlantic Books, 2020.
Identifiers: LCCN 2020005404 (print) | LCCN 2020005405 (ebook) | ISBN
  9781623174071 (trade paperback) | ISBN 9781623174088 (ebook)
Subjects: LCSH: Older men--Psychology. | Self-help techniques.
Classification: LCC HQ1090 .R513 2020 (print) | LCC HQ1090 (ebook) | DDC
  646.7/9--dc23
LC record available at https://lccn.loc.gov/2020005404
LC ebook record available at https://lccn.loc.gov/2020005405

1 2 3 4 5 6 7 8 9 KPC 25 24 23 22 21 20

This book includes recycled material and material from well-managed forests. North Atlantic Books is committed to the protection of our environment. We print on recycled paper whenever possible and partner with printers who strive to use environmentally responsible practices.

This book is dedicated to all aging men and the people who love them

Acknowledgments

I would first like to thank my literary agent, Barbara Lowenstein, for her inspiration and encouragement to write this book. Left to my own devices, it might not have happened. Tim McKee, publisher of North Atlantic, played an outsized role in bringing this book to fruition—not only as the final decision maker in accepting the book, but also by devoting his time and energy as primary editor during its writing. I would also like to thank acquisitions editors Keith Donnell and Pam Berkman, production editor Trisha Peck, copyeditor Jennifer Eastman, and all the people on the production team at North Atlantic Books. They included me and consulted with me every step of the way—an author's dream!

Many people contributed valuable content to the book and made it come alive through their anecdotes, stories, professional advice, strategic direction, and editorial suggestions. My heartfelt thanks to all of them: Marc Agronin, Ralph Bragg, Peter Coyote, Scott Davis, Michael Denneny, Cathy Dykes, Bruce Fortin, John Grubb, Matt Herron, Jack Maslow, Ruth Palmer, Rico Provasoli, Josh Rothenberg, Sam Salkin, Alix Salkin, Jay Vogt, and Angela Winter. Each of you helped make the book wiser and stronger.

Finally, thanks to my wife, Amy—my first and best editor—for patiently reading the whole manuscript several times and suggesting improvements large and small that I would never otherwise have discovered.

Contents

Foreword

I was young once, virile, sure of myself, physically powerful, quick witted, confident, and by my own measure, successful. Now I am seventy-eight, en route to seventy-nine. My feet are permanently asleep from neuropathy affecting my balance. In certain instances, my hands tremble. There's no question of regaining physical vigor or the sexual confidence of my youth. I forget names and occasions with increasing frequency. I am not alone.

My friend and (full disclosure) my Zen teacher for over a dozen years, Lew Richmond, wrote this book for people like me, people being ratcheted forward toward passage on a train that never returns and from which no one escapes. There is a physical element to aging, but the most challenging part may be the mental component. It is this that Lew and this book intend to help us with.

Lew has spent his entire adult life in intimate contact with his own mind. He spent his young manhood living in a Zen Buddhist monastery and went on to found his own software business. During his active career as a Zen teacher, he counseled many people and bore intimate witness to their suffering and confusion. He nearly died in his early fifties and spent weeks in a coma. His recovery took several grueling years. All of which is to assert that he has lived deeply, suffered, and lived to mine the rich veins of wisdom from his experiences.

I can't think of a more perfect person to write a book like this. I have lost track of the number of times during my apprenticeship when Lew—always deeply compassionate, always looking at things clearly—dissipated my confusion, anger, and suffering of one sort of another with a few well-chosen words. Five years after our work together drew to a close, I still call Lew from time to time for his valuable clarity, subtlety, and unfailing compassion.

As my entire generation moves toward its end, I can't think of a more helpful, necessary book. Doctors can help us with our physical suffering but not with the mental suffering that accompanies the loss of power, authority, and meaningfulness—along with the physical decay—that are the final hurdles of human life. We are all dying, and our only viable option is to strive to die well. *Dying well* means, first and foremost, accepting what is happening to us without evasion or excuse. It means trusting that the human body, over millions of years, has learned how to die and will do it quite naturally. It is our egos, our illusions of a separate, graspable, identifiable self that must learn to face and accept the inevitable declines and losses if we are to end our days with joy, dignity, acceptance, and the internal freedom to step aside from our own limited distractions and concerns and not miss the miracle that we participate in until our very last breath.

This book will help you. Lew will show you how, as he's showed me. This is something we *can* do, but in order to do it, we must accept what appears to be so difficult for us—loss, weakness, and disappearance. It *can* be done, and there are legions of elder exemplars to demonstrate how. Lew offers a calm and systematic framework and practice to help you get the most out of your life *right now!* There is no such thing as dying. We are either alive or dead, and while we're alive, we're participating in a miraculous, star-lit universe. Why miss a second of it? Why not learn to love our growing old?

—Peter Coyote

Actor, writer, Zen priest

Author of *Sleeping Where I Fall*
and *The Rainman's Third Cure*

1

INTRODUCTION

As I began writing this book, my wife Amy and I were getting ready to move from the house where we had lived for thirty years and find a smaller home to retire in. I was seventy-one, she was seventy-four. Our reasons for moving were partly financial. The tech boom in San Francisco had boosted our home value, and if we moved just thirty-five miles north, we could harvest our home equity and live in semiretirement more comfortably. But there was another reason for moving. Our house had lots of stairs. Amy had injured her knee recently, and while my legs were still good, we were only one broken ankle or hip replacement away from not being able to negotiate those stairs.

In other words, we were aging. The objective facts of our situation were easy to grasp and made a lot of sense. But there was an emotional component to our decision to move—emotions connected to growing older—that those facts did not capture. These emotions were bittersweet for me. On the one hand, we were excited about moving to a new house, a new town, making new friends, engaging in new activities. On the other hand, we were divesting ourselves of possessions—books, art, furniture, photographs, vinyl records, our son's Lego collection, which we were storing for him for when he had his own children—each of which carried its own memories and emotions of an earlier time.

I was surprised by how strongly these emotions moved me. I was also forced to realize that our new house was likely to be our last house. We would grow old together there and become infirm there. And some day—not for a long time, I hoped—one of us would die there, leaving the other alone. These thoughts evoked strong emotions in me—a feeling of poignancy and sadness. It may be a stereotype to say that men don't easily sense or express their emotions. At least for me at that moment, that stereotype was not really true. However, as the following story illustrates, sometimes the stereotype is true.

Mike was playing golf with three of his friends. One of them, a man named Al, casually mentioned that he had just separated from his wife.

"How do you feel about that?" Mike asked him.

"Feel?" Al said, taken aback. "Mike, what the hell are you talking about?"

What indeed was Mike talking about? How is it that Al, an intelligent, mature man, didn't know how to answer Mike's question? Was it really true that Al didn't understand what the word *feel* means?

The exploration of feeling is one of the reasons I wrote this book, along with the many other aspects of aging that rise up in our inner lives as men that we are ordinarily reluctant to talk about. Actually, I doubt that Al didn't know what Mike was talking about. I think he knew. He just didn't want to go there, to reveal to another man something painful about his inner life. Given a different circumstance or environment, Al might indeed have opened up about how he felt.

You could say I'm writing this book for Al, for Mike, for you and me, and for all the men negotiating the last third of their lives who know intellectually that they are getting older, but aren't sure how they feel about it or what to do about those feelings.

This is my second book on aging. The first one, *Aging as a Spiritual Practice: A Contemplative Guide to Growing Older and Wiser* was published in 2012. In that year I hosted a series of one-day discussion workshops on aging. I typically began these sessions by going around the circle and having people introduce themselves. Typically, the attendees were two-thirds women, one-third men. We began by giving a short statement about our concerns about aging.

Edwin was the first to speak up. "I'm sixty-four, still working. No plans to retire anytime soon." He paused. "The truth is, I haven't thought much about aging. I don't feel old. I'm healthy, happily married, doing all the right things—I eat right, work out, take my meds. When I saw the notice for this group, I thought, *Hey, maybe I should start thinking about getting old.* It's out there, just over the horizon. And whenever I think about it, I picture a kind of dark cloud hanging out there, a rain cloud that hasn't hit yet, but is going to. I'm here to find out more."

A few more men spoke, and then a man introduced himself as Len and simply said, "I'm a retired teacher." Then he paused. It seemed as though Len was going to say more, but he did not. He looked tense.

For the next hour, members of the group engaged in a lively discussion about aging—their concerns about it and what it meant to them. Len, however, said nothing. He just stared at the floor.

Finally, I asked him if he had anything he wanted to say.

"Oh, yeah," he said. "I could say something. I could say a lot of things."

The group waited while Len prepared to speak.

"Yeah, I used to teach English as a second language," Len said finally. "To all kinds of people. Immigrants from all over the world. Latinos who had lived here for a while and wanted to improve their English. College students from abroad. Actually, I was a lot more than just an English teacher. I was a mentor for my students. They were all working hard, struggling to fit in. Finding ways to improve themselves. They were such impressive people. And I was their coach, their guide, the key to their American dream. Those students loved me, and I loved them. Those students were my life."

Len's voice started to shake. "And then the school district came back and told me there were budget cuts. They had to take a look at all the staff, especially ones close to retirement. Like I'm fifty-eight. Close to retirement?" He laughed harshly. "I got the ax. Just like that.

"Like I said, those students were my life," Len repeated. "They were like my kids, every one of them. I'm divorced. No kids of my own. Just like that, I'm gone." Len threw up his hands. "So what am I supposed to do now? Just lie down and die?"

The group was stunned. No one had anything to say. Finally, I said, "That's a pretty tough story, Len. I don't know exactly what to say to you right at this moment, but I can say that there are definitely many things you can do besides lie down and die. That's why we're all here, to talk about that."

Len glanced at me briefly. He threw his hands up again, but this time the gesture felt like, *Ok, I'm listening.*

Men like Edwin and Len—along with their wives, partners, lovers, and companions—need more than just vague intimations or bursts of anger. They need a guide. That's what my book *Aging as a Spiritual Practice* was, but from comments, reviews, and correspondence, I think the majority of its readers were women. I heard from some men who had read it, but more who had bought it for their aging mothers. On the whole, men didn't see the book as a guide written for them. In retrospect, this is not surprising. In researching that book, I talked with many medical and mental health professionals. They all said that men and women approach the issue of aging differently. Women tend to think and talk about aging more readily—especially when they are with their women friends.

Though men's and women's experience of aging are similar in some ways, this book focuses on the ways in which men's aging is different—issues such as identity, virility, emotion, and communication. I hope that in the course of the book, male readers will come to see that aging is not something to avoid or conquer, but an experience to be explored and understood. I think aging for men can be seen not as an unpleasant condition to be endured, but as a kind of heroic journey—perhaps the most important such journey of our lives. And while the book speaks to men, it includes viewpoints and topics of interest to women too. Men's spouses and partners are often the best source of information about what is really going on with them. I also want to acknowledge the experience of gay men, whose loved ones are other men and whose aging issues may coalesce around somewhat different concerns.

Aging is a two-faced coin. On one side is loss—loss of virility, strength, power, possibility, opportunity, and health. On the other side is transformation and growth. This transformation is not an intellectual concept. It is not something that can be grasped merely through reading or thinking. The aging journey is emotional; it happens in the realm of feeling.

Some people ask me, "Why write a book on aging? Do we need to be told how to age? After all, aging is not something we learn how to do. Aging just happens to us, and we deal with it, right?" Well, perhaps so, but there is a lot of territory included in the phrase "deal with it." In spite of what is covered in men's health magazines, aging includes considerably more than a good diet, listening to your doctor, and getting enough exercise. There is an *inner* aspect of aging—a quality of personal growth and development— that many of us may not be noticing or tending to. This is what I call "conscious aging," and it is not something we are typically taught how to do. Perhaps in traditional societies the stages and practices of aging were supplied by culture and tradition. But in today's modern societies there is little culture and tradition around aging. You just do it like any other tedious chore. If anything, our society is youth oriented and tends to look away from the needs and feelings of older people.

There are few books about conscious aging for men, and as a general rule, men tend not to buy or read books in the "self-help" category. As one bookstore owner told me, laughing, "Men don't read books unless they are about sex or money."

I replied, "Okay, fine. Both of those are topics that are quite relevant for aging. I'll be sure to include them."

And I will. But the deepest reason I am writing this book is because, as a seventy-two-year-old man who has survived two life-threatening illnesses and who is coming to the end of his active work life, I have searched for that one good book that can speak to me about the challenges of my life as an aging man, and I haven't been able to find it. So, I have written a book that I would like to read, and because I think it might help me, my hope is that it will help you too.

Fears

One fact about aging that we would rather not have other men know is that we have fears. Paula Spencer Scott, writing for the online magazine *Caring* has identified five fears that men have about aging: impotence, weakness, retirement and irrelevance, loss of independence, and losing your mind (or having your wife or partner lose theirs).

Probably all five of these fears could be summarized under the single term *weakness*. As men, we don't like feeling weak. There are many kinds of weakness, but when Paula Scott spoke of weakness, she was referring to actual physical weakness: loss of physical strength, not being able to lift a heavy box or a bag of groceries—or in extreme cases, not being able to even stand or walk.

I experienced this myself at the age of fifty-two when I was struck down with a life-threatening brain infection and awoke from a two-week coma so weak I was unable to lift my head or turn over in bed. It took me two months of intensive rehab before I was able to walk. My doctors and family were overjoyed that I had not died, that I wasn't blind or paralyzed, and that I had all my mental faculties. But I was crushed. I was so weak! I had gone from being a high-functioning, capable man to being what seemed to me practically a vegetable. I felt ashamed and humiliated, not able even to go to the bathroom or brush my teeth without help.

I will be discussing all five fears that Paula Scott listed in the course of this book. But more importantly, I will make the case that—however many fears we have—*it is okay to be afraid*. In the aging journey, fear can be our guide and friend. It can help us surmount obstacles such as loss, anxiety, and depression and help us see where we can renew our life and start fresh on new ground.

Emotion, Intuition, and Deep Mind

One of the underlying themes of this book is that the real work of aging—the aspect of aging that can be positive and transformative—is *emotional* and *intuitive*. Of course, our intellect can manage some of the outer challenges of aging—exercise, diet, medicine, physical checkups, and so forth. But the real drama of aging, the domain in which all the important changes happen, is in the realm of our emotions. It's how we *feel* about aging, more than what we think about it, that really matters. That said, it is sometimes hard for us men to access how we really feel about aging—especially when it comes to those five fears.

I have already mentioned that men appear to be less emotional than women. As the story about Mike and Al demonstrates, many men do have a harder time easily accessing how they feel about something. This may be partly because of our early socialization as young boys not to show our feelings or insecurities. Some researchers think this reticence may also be neurological. It is not true for all men. There is undoubtedly a bell curve of emotional availability, and each of us has a place on that curve.

The stories and anecdotes in this book about men of various ages and walks of life will explore that range. Many of these men are just like you, with the same concerns and questions about aging that you have.

Much of the material online and in print magazines written for men about aging falls into one of two categories—it is either practical but superficial (five tips for how to feel ten years younger now!) or health oriented. This book takes a different approach. I hope that you already know—or can find out—practical information about how to stay healthy and energetic as you grow older. But there is a whole other dimension to aging—the *inner* dimension—that isn't about hints and tips, diets, exercise, or supplements. This inner dimension is happening beneath the surface of our life, like a subterranean river that flows beneath ordinary consciousness. It might surface occasionally in our dreams, our anxieties, and our random thoughts, but to really enter that river and navigate it well requires a specialized tool—the tool of intuition.

Intuition

We have various names for intuition, such as a *hunch, guess,* or *gut feeling.* Sometimes we personalize an intuition by calling it *lady luck.* In business and politics, people speak of a man as a *gut player,* meaning he follows his hunches. In fact, intuition is simply a core faculty of the human mind, one that we use all the time. It used to be thought that women were more intuitive than men—hence the terms *lady luck* or *woman's intuition*. Recent research—for example, in the books *Gut Feelings* by Gerd Gigerenzer, or *Blink* by Malcolm Gladwell—has proved that this is not true. There is no real gender difference. Men can be as intuitive as women, though they may not notice their intuitive insights with the same ease that women do.

The emerging field of intuition research has also identified three characteristics of intuition. It is quick (three times faster than ordinary thinking), it operates outside of conscious awareness, and it needs little information from the outside world to make its decisions. Intuition seems to reside in a much older part of the brain than thinking does. Intuition developed when a quick reaction to a threat meant the difference between life and death.

Imagine one of our distant ancestors—one who looked more like a chimpanzee than a modern human, perhaps—foraging for food on the savannah. He hears a rustling in the bushes. What is it? It could be a lion! Faster than he can think about it, he leaps for the nearest tree and clambers up to safety. This is roughly how researchers picture intuition's original function.

We still use intuition that way today. When we cross the street to avoid a dark alley, choose which grocery line to stand in, or change lanes in traffic, we are using intuition. Sports is another field that is highly intuitive. Think of a running back weaving downfield or a basketball player driving to the basket. Often, after a game, a reporter will ask an athlete how he managed a particular move or shot. The athlete's answer can sometimes sound vague—not because he doesn't know exactly what he did, but because, being intuitive, his move wasn't really conscious or coming from thinking. Even when intuition is not reacting in the moment, it is watching vigilantly in the background, alert for opportunities or dangers.

Intuition also has an important role to play in aging. You may only think about aging occasionally, when something—like seeing your face in the morning mirror—brings it to your attention. But intuition is tuned into aging all the time. It knows exactly how old you are, it knows all about the subtle changes in your body and mental functioning. When it comes to aging, intuition is your inner hourglass.

Remember, though, that intuition is unconscious. We aren't usually aware of it, but intuition has ways of letting you know indirectly what it is up to. It does not use words or concepts; that is the language of thinking, and intuition is not about thinking. Intuition sends us its messages and insights through a physical sensation, an emotion, or an image—the way a dream does. When we are overly focused on what we think and aren't tuned to body and emotion, we miss the message intuition is trying to tell us. Intuition knows things that we may not be consciously tracking. With regard to aging, intuition knows that we are slowing down and that our bodies are changing in myriad ways. It also knows that someday we will die, and all the things that we love and cherish will vanish. That's not something we like to think about, but at all times, day or night, intuition is aware of that.

In short, intuition is where the deepest truths of your life reside.

This book provides tools to help you get in touch with your intuition, become comfortable with it, and trust it. In our premodern past, intuition helped with survival and essential wisdom. It was embedded in legend, myth, and religious ritual and was honored through those expressions. Today, in our fast-paced modern world, driven by technology, social media, and the energies and interests of youth, it is easy to lose that connection. In premodern societies there were specific roles and responsibilities that elder men grew into and were respected for in ensuring the well-being of themselves and the community. For example, male elders had a role in mentoring younger men and helping them know the right way to live. Elders also held the collective wisdom of the community, such as where to find game and when the rains would come—knowledge that was often critical for survival.

This male mentoring is not unique to human beings. In the 1990s, young male elephants were killing white rhinos in a game preserve.[1] They were also tearing up trees, pushing down fences, and harassing the other elephants. The park rangers called in an elephant expert who simply said, "Get an older bull elephant. That will take care of the problem."

The rangers did; they brought in an older male elephant and had him mingle with the younger males. The older male didn't seem to do much except graze quietly and keep to himself. But like magic, the younger males calmed down. The problems disappeared.

Because we no longer live in small, intact social groups like these elephants did, men may not be aware that we have an important role to play as elders, exemplars, and guides for the next generation to follow. I hope this book will help us remember our responsibilities as elders.

The Eight Stages of Life

I have designed this book to be light on theory, with more emphasis on anecdotes, experiences, and practices. That said, there is some descriptive and analytic literature on the stages of a man's life. *The Seasons of a Man's Life*, a 1986 book by psychologist Daniel Levinson, studied the maturing stages of a man, from boyhood to old age. Robert A. Johnson, eminent Jungian analyst, wrote a book in the 1980s entitled *He*, in which he uses the legend of the knight Parsifal and his search for the Holy Grail to epitomize a man's lifelong search for meaning, wisdom, and his rightful role in family and society. The theory that I myself have found most useful is the system of eight life stages developed in the 1950s by psychoanalyst Erik Erikson.

I studied with Erikson when I was in college and loved the way he spoke outside the customs of usual academic thinking. When the class studied old age, he had us read and discuss Shakespeare's *King Lear*.

King Lear hated being old; eventually his fear of aging and his distress at losing all of his royal powers and prerogatives drove him mad, though only temporarily. By the end of the play, he finally comes to terms with all the profound and positive ways his life had changed and understood that his greatest treasure was not his power and possessions as king, but the love of Cordelia, his youngest daughter.

King Lear's epiphany and transformation is a timeless lesson in what we need to learn as men. Each of us, in his own way, inwardly imagines he is the king of his own life and domain, but as life wends its way to its end, it is whom he loves and who loves him that really matters most. That is one of the key themes this book will explore.

Erikson divided the arc of human life into eight developmental stages, beginning with infancy and ending in old age. He called the last stage *ego integrity*; this is the stage when, like Lear, we have come at last to fully accept the life we have lived in all its ups and downs, its triumphs and tragedies. Erikson called the stage just before it *generativity*. Generativity—spanning roughly the ages thirty to sixty-five—meant for Erikson a time of growth and adult maturity when a person contributes to society through children and family, career and livelihood. Ego integrity, in contrast, is a time to come to terms with the life we have lived and realize that in spite of our regrets and paths not taken, we can say, like King Lear, that we are content with the life we have lived and are ready to simply love and be loved.

For a man, successfully negotiating the challenges of generativity and ego integrity means dealing with issues of identity, virility, and power. As life unfolds, a man needs to continue to renew his answer to the question, *what does it mean to be a man?* The answer will vary depending on how he was raised, how he imagines his identity, and how comfortable he is looking within himself. Rather than Ego Integrity—a technical psychological term—I prefer the term deep acceptance. I think deep acceptance captures in ordinary language the feeling of what Erikson meant.

Deep Mind Reflections

In order to enhance your capacity for intuition and deep emotion, I have created a series of imaginative exercises to help you to explore these inner resources—one or two at the end of each chapter. I call these exercises *deep mind reflections*. I came up with the term *deep mind* because it points to the part of your mind where intuition resides and also because it helps engender the deep acceptance of which Erikson speaks. Deep mind is not some magical or exotic place; it is simply the part of your mind that becomes visible when you are quiet. I also thought of calling this realm *quiet mind*. You can think of deep mind as the "quiet you." Deep mind includes intuition, but it also includes imagination and memory. Like intuition, it is always watching and waiting, just under the surface of your busy, thinking mind, ready to help you when you need it, and ready to invest any situation with deeper insight.

Deep mind is just another aspect of you yourself. Just as you can talk to yourself, you can talk to your deep mind. You can invoke it, raise it up, and ask it questions. Talking to deep mind is just another way of talking to yourself, and I have provided a method that allows you to do that.

Deep mind knows many things about you that you may not always be aware of; for example, it knows all about your aging. It knows how old you are and remembers the days, weeks, months, and years that got you here. You may not want to dwell on the feeling of time passing—there is often some sadness to it—but deep mind is not perturbed. It is always looking out for you, always ready to help you. You just have to quiet down and listen.

The next chapter will show you how.

2

GUIDE TO DEEP MIND REFLECTION

Throughout this book, I offer a series of deep mind reflections—one or two at the end of each chapter. The purpose of these exercises in creative imagination is to put you in touch with your deep mind. Deep mind is a type of intuition, and it can reveal new possibilities and fresh perspectives. You may or may not be familiar with this kind of introspection, where you turn your attention inward to observe what is going on inside. If you are—through meditation or some other kind of inner work—then these deep mind reflections might be familiar to you. And if you aren't, that's fine too. The reflections are not difficult, even for a beginner. They are a little like daydreaming—which is something you probably do regularly anyway.

Deep mind is my term for the not-unfamiliar state of mind you enter whenever your mind is quiet—a mental state in which ideas and concepts recede into the background, and emotions and feelings can come forward. A deep understanding of aging is not, in the end, about concepts and ideas as much as it is about emotions and feelings. These deep mind reflections can help you tune in to those feelings.

Once I have explained in detail the stages of the reflection, I will have more to say about related topics, such as the difference between thinking and feeling, the meaning of the term *unconscious* and its relationship to deep mind, and the principle I call *every breath, new chances*. Finally, I will conclude with an example of myself doing a deep mind reflection.

Incidentally, I encourage women readers of this book not to skip over this chapter. Learning about deep mind can help you better understand the men in your lives and come up with better ways of communicating with them. To that end, I devote chapter 10, "What Women Know," to describing the experiences of a number of women I interviewed about the aging men in their lives. At the end of that chapter there is a deep mind reflection specifically designed for women readers to do.

Stages of Deep Mind Reflection

Each reflection is organized around four principles or stages. The first is becoming quiet, resting the mind and body so that you can tune in to your inner "radio channel." The second is focusing on a keyword. In this chapter I will use *aging* as the keyword; in other chapters I will suggest other keywords. The third is an image or picture that expresses or illustrates the keyword. I call this the *key image*. I will suggest some images to try, but I encourage you to pick an image from your own experience and imagination.

As an example of how that would work, after you bring up the keyword *aging*, you could picture the grey hair you see when you look in the mirror each morning. That is a key image that matches up well with the keyword *aging*.

The fourth stage is more open ended and is really the heart of the reflection. This stage takes your use of imagination still further. After becoming quiet, focusing on your keyword and your key image, you then simply open yourself up to all the places your imagination might take you, all the byways of deep mind that you might want to explore.

This is where your intuition really takes the lead. The keyword and the key image are merely a device to unlock your intuition, and once that door is opened, intuition can lead you still further, on an interior adventure into the terrain of your deeper self. And in describing each reflection, I will often include an example of what happened to me when I did the reflection myself. That way my experience can offer another clue for how to negotiate the exercise yourself.

Deep mind reflection is a little like free association; it also has some quality of daydreaming. However, my principal inspiration in developing these reflections was a type of Buddhist inquiry in which you explore a question from all angles while letting your attention wander freely. The core purpose of these reflections is to engender *conscious aging*—to connect your conscious mind with the feelings and emotions about aging that lie just beneath the surface of consciousness, like trout in a quiet eddy in a rushing stream.

Beginning the Reflection

The reflection begins by sitting quietly and clearing the mind. There are many ways to do this. These days, it is important to prepare by first spending some time away from all electronic devices—smartphones, laptops, televisions, or iPads. These machines distract the nervous system from being able to settle down and be quiet.

Next is to find a quiet place to sit, a place free from distractions and from other voices and people. Perhaps there is a place in your home that will do. A place in nature, possibly after a run or walk, is ideal. If you are outside, don't take your smartphone with you, or at least turn it off. We are so wedded to our phones these days that being more than a few feet away causes a mild sense of discomfort and withdrawal. Actually, we live in a world suffused with distractions of all kinds. The first step in actually touching your inner world of aging is to reverse that distraction. Over-fifties are the last generation that will ever remember a time when there were not personal computers.

Perhaps you can think back to a time when you were young and there were no cellphones or computers. Back then—the stone age of the electronic world—it was relatively easy to clear the mind and relax. Now it takes more effort. However, that bygone childhood world innocent of electronic distraction is still a memory you can retrieve and enjoy.

Turning your attention to the ebb and flow of breathing is another good method, one that has now become popular and well known. There are several methods. One method is to pay attention to the subtle sensation at the tip of your nostrils of air flowing in and air flowing out. Another is to put your attention in the center of your body and feel the sensation of breath coming in and filling you, and breath going out and leaving. Some people find it effective to count their breaths, counting each exhale from one to ten and back again. You will know you are ready to begin the reflection when you check in with your inner dialogue and find that it is not saying or thinking much.

Keyword and Key Image

The next step is to settle on a keyword and a key image. At the end of each chapter, I will suggest a keyword or words for you to try. In this chapter, in the example of my own reflection, I use the keyword *aging*. As you tune in to the inner landscape of thinking—where, by now, hopefully there are not too many random thoughts—every so often, like a soft hammer striking a bell, say the keyword silently to yourself: aging. Not too often, perhaps every ten or fifteen seconds, ring that bell: aging. That's it, that's all you need to do. It doesn't matter what else is going on in your mind. The keyword sounds at regular intervals, softly, quietly, without fuss. At this stage you needn't pay attention to the meaning of the keyword. Your deep mind will be awakened by it and will begin to respond to it. Of course, the word *aging* has meaning, and your deep mind is well aware of that meaning. At this point it is just a word: aging.

The key image will typically be something related to the keyword. I will be suggesting some possible images, and you may use those, but the best image is one that comes from your own associations and memories. Don't work too hard to discover an image; let intuition bring one to you. For myself, when I repeat the word *aging*, the image that comes to mind is the head of hair that I see in the mirror each morning, grey going on white. That may not be appropriate for you—for instance, your hair may not yet be grey, or you may be bald. The image doesn't have to be visual; it can be a sound, a touch, even a smell. A physical sensation or condition works for some people. For example, if you are developing arthritis in one knee, your image could be the discomfort in your knee.

So now, each time you "ring" the bell of your keyword, bring up your key image just afterward. You can think of it like an echo of your keyword. In my own example, every so often I would ring the bell of the word *aging*, and follow on with an inner picture of the grey hair I see in the mirror. Aging, grey hair. Aging, grey hair.

New Keywords and Images

As you engage in the process of repetition, your deep mind will be awakened and will begin to participate in the process. At some point either the keyword or the image may spontaneously change. This is your deep mind moving the reflection into its own terrain, following its own inner trajectory. So the word *aging* might turn into *ageist*, bringing up feelings of being discriminated against for being older. Or *aging* could turn into *edgy*; maybe the thought of aging is making your deep mind feel anxious.

In the same way, the image can spontaneously change. Instead of looking at your grey hair in the mirror, for example, your deep mind might hone in on the bags under your eyes. Or you might suddenly see the face of your aged grandfather in the mirror.

You can respond to these shifts in a couple of ways. You could follow them, replacing your keyword or key image with the new ones that have arisen. Or you could simply take note of the shift and return to your original word and image. You can experiment with each of these strategies and see what happens.

Duration and Cautions

There is no set time period that is optimal for the reflection. Generally speaking, you should start with a short period at first—three to five minutes—to accustom yourself to the process. As you become comfortable with it, you can lengthen the time.

For most people the reflection is a benign investigation that helps you know yourself better on the inside. But occasionally, deep mind may take you into territory—particularly with the key image—that you find upsetting. The minute that happens, break off the exercise, and do not return to it until you feel comfortable. And when you do, do not use the same keyword or key image that landed you in uncomfortable terrain.

There are aspects of aging—particularly the physical parts—that are no fun. For example, when older people get together, they can find themselves "playing the organ recital"—that is, speaking about their various ailments, their aches and pains. But aging is also maturity, the fruit and experience of a whole life. That fruit cannot be picked until it is ripe. Younger people, no matter how brilliant their minds or how fertile their imaginations, cannot truly understand what it means to be old. The ripeness of growing older can lead to many surprising and unexpected joys. The reflection can lead you in the direction of some of these and open those possibilities up to you. That is the most important function of the reflection: to get you out of your routines and your well-worn pathways and open up new vistas.

Taking Notes

It is best, particularly at the outset, not to take many notes as the reflection proceeds. You could jot down a word or phrase as you go to help you remember, but as with a dream journal, it usually works best to write down what happened in a session of reflection after it has concluded.

Ending the Reflection

The reflection ends as it begins: clearing your mind of all the words and images that have come to mind, letting your attention focus on the rising and falling of the breath. The reflection is a little like a waking dream—a self-guided daydream, if you will. Once it has ended, it should dissipate. You can make sure it does by turning your attention to a working task that requires all your concentration— checking your email, perhaps, or reading the news. Any notes you have taken will remind you of the significant aspects of the session; you need not make any conscious effort to remember it. Besides, your deep mind will remember it for you. The next time you take up the reflection, deep mind will remember where in the reflection you have been and will remind you of anything it thinks you need to know.

This concludes the how-to guide for doing deep mind reflection. What follows is a discussion of some related topics that can give you a more thorough perspective of what deep mind reflection is and is not, as well as an example from my own experience of how a session of deep mind reflection actually goes.

Thinking and Feeling

Unless we are very quiet, we are always thinking. By *thinking* I mean our moment-to-moment mental activity, which we often experience as a running dialogue of internal speech. But thinking is only one kind of mental activity. The realm of emotion and intuition that exists beneath our inner dialogue is another flavor of mental activity. When we think about aging in our moment-to-moment inner dialogue, it might sound something like this:

Of course I'm growing old; I just had a birthday. So what? I still feel good, I can perform in bed, and I can run a mile in ten minutes. I'm not really old. When I start to get really old, I'll deal with it then. Until then, I don't really want to think about it.

This may or may not be what you really actually say to yourself. Everyone thinks about aging differently. But I have talked to many men who tell themselves some version of this aging story. That kind of thinking about aging is like a casual conversation with ourselves—like talking about sports, work, weekend plans, or the weather. That's our surface mind talking. Meanwhile, underneath all of that, deep mind listens to your chattering like a wise old friend, nodding but not talking, knowing that there is more to your aging story. There are truths about yourself in the realm of feelings and emotions that it would be good for you to know—that you will know when you slow down, become quiet, and hear what deep mind has to say.

In exploring deep mind, it might help to mention the term *unconscious*, since that is a commonly understood psychological concept. The unconscious is that part of the mind that functions outside of ordinary waking awareness. Since we don't directly experience the unconscious, it may seem exotic or mysterious, but there's really nothing mysterious about it. In fact, when you think about it, almost everything that happens throughout your day is unconscious. Our breathing and heartbeats are unconscious; so are our bodily movements such as standing and walking, as well as automated skills such as tying your shoes and driving a car. In fact, almost everything that we do is unconscious except whatever task we are focusing on. If we had to be conscious of everything we do, we would become paralyzed from the overload. Our brain operates on autopilot for most things.

The unconscious is also the storehouse of memory. We have, stored away in our brain, a lifetime of remembered experiences. They are all unconscious until we need to remember something, and then they come up. Because the unconscious knows so much, it can react to situations in ways we are not aware of. For example, when we are in a stressful situation, such as a job interview, our stress reaction happens largely outside of our awareness, which remains focused on the interview itself. It is only after the interview is done and we are in the elevator that we become conscious of our sweaty palms and beating heart.

Another function of the unconscious is dreaming. Dreams are unlike waking experience. Dreams are not linear; they are seemingly illogical and fragmentary, and they occur mostly as a sequence of pictures and images rather than words.

So deep mind is not really unconscious in the usual meaning of that term. Deep mind is part of waking mind, although it may draw upon unconscious memories and emotions. Deep mind is a mind free from distraction, inner dialogue, and random thinking. What deep mind brings into awareness, when you are quiet, are thoughts and feelings that you want and need to know. Deep mind is the part of yourself that cares deeply for you and wants the best for you. We all have that part of ourselves within us. It is that kindly grandparent who loves to watch us play and wants to see us grow. In the case of these deep mind reflections about aging, deep mind wants to see us age well and with dignity. Deep mind, in that sense, is always looking out for us.

So these deep mind reflections are a kind of reverie, invoked and loosely guided by a keyword and one or more images. The reflection is not therapy, nor is it self-hypnosis. It is something that you probably already do from time to time, whenever you are working on a life problem or seeking a solution for a vexing question. These deep mind reflections turn that familiar problem-solving process into an investigative tool.

Aging is somewhat different from an ordinary life problem. For one thing, while some aspects of aging are personal, others are universal. In other words, how you experience your own aging may be particular to your character and life experience, but at the same time, everyone—in fact, every living thing—ages. Our experience of aging actually starts early, as soon as we are old enough to think and talk and know our age. Young children are quite aware of their age, and if you ask them how old they are, they will say with great emphasis and precision, "Three and three quarters." Children want to be older, bigger, and grown up. This yearning to be older continues well into adulthood as we attain the milestones of maturity—having our first romantic relationship, graduating from high school or college, getting our first job or apartment, marrying, having children.

It is only somewhat past the midpoint of life that this calculus slowly shifts—imperceptibly at first, and then more noticeably. At some point we realize that, all things considered, we would like to be younger, not older. The actual age when this happens varies. It could be when you are in your forties, fifties, or even sixties. But whenever it happens, there is some noticeable point where the seesaw of our life tilts in the other direction, and we begin to feel some regret at the passing of years. And even before your conscious mind notices, your deep mind has taken note and has started to send signals in your emotional reactions and dreams, signals that say, "Hello. You are starting to get old."

Deep mind reflection is a method to tune in to the radio channels of those signals, pick them up, understand what they mean, and make them conscious.

Every Breath, New Chances

A Buddhist teacher once said to me, "Every breath, new chances." He told me that this principle had helped guide him through difficulties in his own life. When I asked him to explain this phrase more deeply, he replied that it meant three things: everything changes; every change can be an opportunity; and sitting quietly and sensing the breath helps those opportunities to reveal themselves.

Every breath, new chances means that no situation is fixed and that any situation can change—sometimes for the worse, but often for the better. Life is full of surprises. This is a core Buddhist principle and also a psychological one. A psychiatrist friend once told me that the advice he gives to patients who feel stuck is, "There is always something you can do." This is similar to what my Buddhist teacher said. The challenge is discovering what that "something" is.

Every breath, new chances could also be a description of intuition and how deep mind reflection works. The reflection uses the resource of intuition to help us see a situation with fresh eyes and with new perspectives. It helps us tune in to our gut feelings about where to go and what to do, as we journey into unknown territory, a place where there are no marked trails and we have to scour the landscape for clues.

Aging is a journey like that—a decades-long adventure with many byways and surprises. It has an itinerary that is partly known and partly unknown. To some extent there is a map—we can partly see where we are going as we age—but the map is not complete. Some parts of the map are filled in, some parts are unclear, and some seem to be blank. Deep mind can help us fill in this map as we go. When we come to a fork in the road—when, for example, we are deciding whether or not to retire and what to do afterward—intuition and the principle of *every breath, new chances* can help us decide what is best.

The journey of aging doesn't go on forever, of course; it comes to an end when life ends. But death and dying are not the focus of this book. My interest is in helping you negotiate your living journey, so that long before the end approaches, you can say, as, "This life I have lived is good. I leave with no regrets."

In the last chapter I told the story of Al, who mentioned during a golf game that he had just separated from his wife. When Al was asked, "How do you feel about that?" Al replied to his friend, "Feel? Mike, what the hell are you talking about?"

Al is someone who probably doesn't spend much time focusing on how he feels about things. Instead, he keeps his attention turned outward, to the events going on around him. However, his response clues us in to the fact that, whether he was aware of it or not, Al was feeling plenty inside. He just didn't want to deal with it.

Remember Len, the English teacher who was forced into early retirement and said, "What am I supposed to do now? Lie down and die?" Len was feeling a powerful emotion—anger—so he undoubtedly knew how he felt, but he didn't have a method ready at hand to deal with that anger constructively.

Deep mind reflection is a form of questioning that uses the imagination as well as intuition. The reflection encourages you to ask, *Now that I am focused on my inner life, where is that leading me? What is it telling me? How can it help me?*

My Experience

Let me now share with you my own experience of a deep mind reflection. Even though I am the one describing the reflection to you, that does not mean I have any special expertise in doing it. I am just another aging man with my particular life history and aging story.

I began with the keyword *aging*. When I called to mind an image, I first thought of the white hair I see in the mirror, but then my thoughts shifted to a gnarled tree along the creek side path where my wife and I walk every morning. This tree is not devoid of foliage—it is not dead—but not all of its branches are leafed out. It is like a man who is balding; he once had a full head of black hair. Now his hair is grey, thinning on the sides, and he has only a few wisps on top. This tree has been through painful times, I can see. One of its main branches is cracked and broken, as though at one time it had been struck by lightning. With my duo of life-threatening illnesses, that is like me too. I have been struck and hit hard. The tree and I are both still standing, however.

Aging, aging. I repeat the word to myself with the image of the gnarled tree in my mind's eye. On the one hand, I am so happy to still be here. Were it not for high-tech medicine, talented doctors, and a prompt arrival at the emergency room just as I was falling into unconsciousness, I would not be here. On the other hand—and the image of the balding tree hits home here—I will not be here for all that much longer.

Aging, aging. I'm hearing echoes of another, related word: *ancient.* I would not like to think of myself as ancient, not yet anyway. But there is the biblical phrase, "ancient of days." This phrase was used in the Book of Daniel as a title of God; in religious art, the ancient of days is pictured as an old man. There is a famous etching by William Blake of the ancient of days as an old man with a white beard. Although ancient of days in a biblical sense has a specific meaning as God, it could, in ordinary language, also just mean an old man. Like me, like you. When I count my life in days, rather than years, there have been an uncountable cascade of days, most of which I cannot remember. I imagine that's another reading of ancient of days.

A child is not an ancient of days; he or she is fresh of days. A friend of told me this story: a couple was visiting them for dinner, accompanied by their young son, who was about three. Soon after they arrived, they realized that they didn't have the house gift they had brought—a bottle of wine. Somehow it had been left behind.

"Where's that wine?" the father kept repeating, rummaging through the tote bag they had brought.

Suddenly the three-year-old piped up. "I don't know," he said gaily. "I'm new."

Once I too was new. Once we all were new. But now we are all tarnished and dented from long use, like old metal teapots. We have become ancients of days, in the ordinary language sense.

Ancient, ancient. The word changes again in my mind, while the image of the gnarled tree drifts in and out of awareness. *Ancient* becomes *patient.*

Immediately I understand that the word *patient* has two meanings. One meaning is to be patient, willing to let things unfold in their own time, like each day, like a tree in every season and weather. The other meaning, more ominous, is to be *a* patient, as in a hospital—a patient such as I have been many times in my life, and such as I may be once again, when the end is near.

Aging, ancient, patient. That is the trajectory my mind has taken me in language. It's a microcosm of the aging journey, happening in just a few minutes of placid reflection. Your journey, your image, your words will be different, as they should be.

How do I feel when I ponder my own deep mind reflection? A mixture of things. I feel a bit somber; sometimes aging can feel that way. On the other hand, my deep mind took me on a bit of an adventure—aging, ancient, patient—and I feel that deep mind is looking out for me, taking care of me like that kind old grandfather. That is the job our deep mind has, to do the best it can to look out for us as we wander about in our awakened day. There is a dream the unconscious dreams behind the scrim of what we do each day, and that dream sustains us, like a secret food. Each man who ages can be nourished by this secret food. That is one message of this book. Whether we engage the aging journey consciously or not, whether we listen to what our deep mind is trying to tell us or not, we each have a kind old grandfather who helps us along.

When I think that way, then my feeling about my reflection is good. I dipped into my sustaining dream, and said hello to my kind old grandfather.

3

VIRILITY AND POWER

Beginning in midlife, men start to worry about the decline of their various masteries and abilities—including sexual ability. Because virility and power are core elements of male identity, their waning—however gradual—can trigger deep anxiety. Virility means, besides the ability to perform sexually, the power to influence and control your destiny—at work, at home, and in relationships. Men want to be in control, and any loss of control—whether physical, sexual, work related, or relational—is a challenge. In her article in *Caring*, Paula Spencer Scott says that "the prospect of impotence was scarier than cancer or death to readers of a popular men's magazine." I don't know that this is true for all men; there is certainly a range of reactions. But the reference to "cancer or death" indicates how closely sexual performance and core identity are linked.

Scott also wrote about the fear of weakness in men as they age. She was referring not to metaphorical weakness, but actual physical weakness. She expresses it this way: "If I can't lift things, what kind of man am I?"

Speaking of lifting, one humbling lesson I learned about packing everything up and moving out of our home is that moving means lifting. And lifting means coming to terms with how much I don't have a young body anymore. That was where the decision to move and the hard fact of being old unhappily intersected. Not being as strong as I would like in one insignificant way (lifting boxes) made me feel not as strong in every significant way.

I injured my back decades ago and haven't been able to lift anything heavy since. Not being able to lift the moving boxes was just another insult in a lifelong decline. Just after I first injured myself, I remember feeling embarrassed when another man would ask me to help him move a piece of furniture, and I would have to demur. What was I embarrassed about? What difference did it make what the other man thought of me? But in my mind, there was the thought, *I'm weak! Can't let it show.*

Fortunately, after a few years and a few more careless reinjuries, I concluded that taking care of my back was more important than avoiding embarrassment.

Sexual Performance

Psychologically speaking, virility, strength, and power are all closely related. The two meanings of the word *impotence* capture this connection. In a sexual context, it means the inability to perform, but as a general term, it means powerlessness or weakness.

Some loss of sexual function as we age is normal. An article in *Sexual Advice Association,* an online magazine, reports that "half of men between the ages of 40 and 70 will experience difficulty attaining and keeping an erection to some degree."[1] Forty years ago, this was a frustrating problem. These days "there is a pill for that"—in fact, several pills, as well as other medical fixes like implants and injections—so erectile dysfunction (ED) is, from a medical or physiological perspective, mostly manageable.

Those pills do not necessarily help with the psychological effects of erectile dysfunction, however. Decline in sexual ability—no matter how you treat it—is still a decline, and emotionally that decline can weigh on men as a more fundamental loss of power and control.

To that point, I read a news report recently that described a new international study conducted across eight countries.[2] The study found that erectile dysfunction is associated with problems on the job and an overall decline in quality of life. The study also found that men suffering from erectile dysfunction were more likely to fall behind at work and become less productive. Erectile dysfunction was also linked to greater rates of staying home from work and working while sick.

"Besides just the workplace," the study said, "erectile dysfunction was found to be associated with higher rates of everyday life activity impairment, and lower overall physical and mental quality of life." Erectile dysfunction is one of the primary ways that our bodies tell us, incontrovertibly, that we are getting older. The real issue, in the end, is not what our knees or our hips or our sexual organs tell us about the impending decline in our powers, but the way in which our identity as a man is tied to those powers. Finding a way to understand our identity outside of the nexus of power and weakness is key to dealing with growing older without difficulty. That shift in identity can lead to a new kind of mastery, one that actually grows stronger, not weaker, with age. Though our bodies may become less powerful with each passing year, a deeper awareness of who we really are can become correspondingly stronger.

Patrick spoke of this shift in his post on my aging blog.

At eighty-seven, I've experienced a decided drop in my libido. My wife and I have found ways to adapt to this—we haven't given up intimacy, but we've come to cherish our moments of closeness, even if they don't lead to climax.

In other areas, I feel as alive as ever. I've taken up the study of the double bass and play in a community orchestra. I continue my seventeen-year adventure of flying gliders cross country and recently went to Lithuania to purchase a new motor glider. Physically, I notice that I don't have the energy reserves I once had, and I usually fit in a half-hour afternoon nap. I exercise daily, work out at a health club at least twice a week, and understand that this regimen is absolutely vital to my continued health as an older man. How do I regard the inevitable diminution of my powers? I look on aging as just another adventure, requiring adaptation as my body and brain change, but I don't dwell much on the future—the present is entirely too interesting.

Kinds of Power

Virility is one kind of power important to men. But for many or most men, power in general is a quality closely tied to their identities. Having power makes us feel respected, valued, and strong. The importance of power in our lives as men may be partly genetic and partly something we learn growing up. My own experience as a boy is illustrative.

As a boy, I was never physically strong, nor was I good at throwing or kicking a ball, arm wrestling, or climbing a rope. Physical education was my most stressful subject, not least because I skipped two grades in elementary school and was small in a class of larger boys. In the 1950s this is what happened to "gifted" children with ambitious parents; my mother and father had no clue that putting me in the seventh grade at the age of ten with a bunch of rough-and-tumble twelve-year-olds was a perfect setup to be bullied. And bullied I was—fairly mildly by today's standards, but bullied nonetheless. I had a quick way with words, though. I chattered my way out of any number of dicey situations with the tough boys. I was also physically quick, with fast reflexes, and handball was the one sport where I could actually keep up and compete. On the playground it was important to be good at *something*, so my handball skills helped.

During my school years, I also discovered that physical strength was not the only kind of power. My verbal quickness did indeed help me avoid fights; that was a kind of power. Sometimes I wanted to be able to fight and actually got into a few minor scuffles until my parents sat me down and informed me that as I was a serious piano student, my hands were valuable, and I was never to raise my fists to anyone again. So my developing male ego never organized itself around physical strength. Instead, I reveled in being known—by the teachers as well as the kids—as one of the smart kids in my high school.

When I came of age as an adult in the "revenge of the nerds" era of the 1970s and 1980s, being smart eventually became a ticket to social status and earning power. I had studied music and philosophy in college—not subjects leading to an impressive paycheck—and after graduation, I spent a decade first in a Christian seminary and then living as a Buddhist monastic. Then I joined the corporate workplace and taught myself how to write software—a skill that in time led to starting my own software business and attaining at least a middling level of earning power, though it was more than I could have imagined during my contemplative Buddhist days.

Still, the old image of myself as a weak, small boy among larger, stronger boys lurked somewhere inside my adult psyche. It wasn't until I started my own software company that I understood the status ladder of men in business. At the lower and middle rungs of the ladder were employees. Certainly, if you were an executive, as I was for a while, you had higher status than clerks and middle managers, but still, you were hired help and could be fired. Next up the ladder were consultants. They worked for themselves—meaning nobody could fire them—and had higher status as independent operators. But highest on the ladder—even if your company had only six employees, as mine did—were business owners. When I went to trade shows to demo my software, my business card said, "Founder and President." People took notice of that. When men at the gym asked me what I did for a living, I could answer "I own a software company" and establish myself at the top of the male status ladder.

Having spent twelve years in a Buddhist retreat community where no one had any income of their own and the only values that mattered were spiritual ones, I could step back and find all these status games rather odd. Because of my Buddhist years, I hadn't entered the workforce until I was thirty-five, yet here I was, ten years later, affecting the status and confidence of a business owner. I appreciated the benefits of that, though in some part of my psyche, I was still back in the Buddhist community, unconcerned about status.

Fast forward thirty-five years, and here I was, retiring from all that, getting ready to move, lifting box after box of give-away books into the car to cart to the library. At first my back rebelled only modestly—a little soreness getting out of bed in the morning. But with each library trip, the soreness got worse, until I was limping around in real pain. My wife took to lifting most of the heavy boxes; I was the semi-invalid. It wasn't like being in the rehab hospital, where I was too weak to turn over in bed. No, but to my male ego, it was still a significant humiliation. Why can't I lift these boxes packed only half-full to keep the weight down? Answer: because I am old.

Old, old, old. My inner critic laughed at me for letting such a small thing bother me. But my eternal inner child—the one who was small and weak and couldn't throw a football—wasn't amused. *I'm not strong; I'll never be strong*, it said. But there was hope: we were moving to a house where there would be no stairs. And once we got there, I promised myself, we will get a local handyman to move whatever heavy objects need to be moved.

The Deeper Meaning of Power

Why are feelings of strength and power so important to us as men? We could speculate that we have evolved that way as protectors of our community and warriors against our enemies. But that's just one kind of explanation. What really matters is who we think we are, and how feelings of power support that.

"That's right," Edward said to me when I asked him what he felt was essential to being a man. "Being a man means having power."

"What kind of power?" I said.

"All kinds," Edward replied. "Money, status, authority, respect, sex—you name it." He paused. "Look, I turned sixty last year. I'm overweight. I'm losing my hair. But I have money, and I'm a successful lawyer. After my divorce I thought, *how is it going to be with women?* But I shouldn't have worried. They're beating down my door, women twenty or thirty years younger. Why? Because I've got the money and the power."

"And you can keep up with these younger women?" I ventured.

Edward nodded. "Sure. Time of my life."

Reflecting on this conversation, I realized how dependent Edward was on all his signifiers of power and how distressed he would be if any of them were to falter.

Edward listed several reasons why power and control are so central to a man's identity—particularly those fifty or older, who were raised and socialized according to the *masculine stereotype,* a topic discussed more fully in the next chapter. Some of these reasons are well established by research, others are more anecdotal and speculative. It is well known that the average male big-company CEO is two or three inches taller than other men in the company.[3] And it is still the case that over 90 percent of Fortune 500 CEOs are men—not women—and in spite of much well-meaning effort, that glass ceiling continues.

After the 2018 midterm elections there were 119 women in the new Congress, the majority of them just elected. This is groundbreaking news only because until now the vast majority of legislators at both the state and federal level have been men. Until recently it was mostly men who have run for office—in other words, it was men who proactively sought positions of power.

Here's another, more subtle, sign of how important and deeply embedded a man's sense of power is. When I left the Buddhist scene for the business world, I noticed that when I walked into a room containing a group of men, I instinctively sized up every man in the room and ranked them in terms of their power. Part of this instinct was strictly physical, that is, I noticed which men were physically larger than I was. Another aspect of my reaction was more intuitive—I found myself sensing through body language which men could be a challenge. As Lyndon Johnson once said, "If you walk into a room, and you can't figure out in five minutes who's for you and who's against you, you don't belong in politics." President Johnson was just giving voice to what I viscerally understood.

I asked a number of men I knew, and after they thought about it, most of them realized they were doing the same thing. Men, it seems, are hard-wired for power comparisons. There was a time, undoubtedly, when such comparisons helped determine the strongest chief or leader. Perhaps in many professional situations, they still do.

Another quality I noticed in myself, especially when I worked as a corporate executive, was my dominating conversational style. I have mentioned that I have always been verbally quick. In business I also learned to cultivate a forceful speaking style. I was good at interrupting and often did to make my point. When I read Deborah Tannen's groundbreaking 1990 book *You Just Don't Understand,* I had a better understanding of what I was doing. Her book was the first of many to document differences between men's and women's speaking styles. Men are more willing to interrupt, often raising their voices to do so—in effect, treating conversations as a kind of competitive sport. Women—partly because they are more sensitive to emotional nuance in a conversation—were typically a half beat behind the men. When they attempted to emulate a male speaking style by raising their voice or interrupting, they were often criticized for being rude or unpleasant—whereas men doing the same thing were seen as capable and effective. Again, conversationally speaking, men seek and wield power.

After my 1999 brain infection, I couldn't walk, stand, eat, or go to the bathroom unaided. For a while I couldn't even speak. For the first time in my life I was dependent on others for nearly all my needs. During my slow recovery, I realized how much of my identity had been tied to being quick, capable, and verbally dominating. It was interesting for me to discover that while I felt ashamed and powerless, the women in my life told me they liked me better this way. "You don't interrupt all the time," they said. "You're actually listening to us for a change."

Even after my "masculine" powers returned, I never forgot how weak I once had been. I also remembered the biggest lesson I learned from that time: people close to me loved me not because of my skills and powers, but simply because of who I was.

A Different Way to Understand Power

Aging includes a loss of power and control, sometimes gradual, sometimes sudden. Rudy, age fifty-six, had been a lifelong athlete: a high-school football and wrestling star, an avid golfer, basketball player, and martial-arts aficionado. After he injured a knee playing basketball, an orthopedic surgeon told him that while he didn't require surgery now, he would at some point and would have to give up all movement sports—permanently. Rudy was devastated.

"So now I'm a vegetable? I have to sit around the house every weekend like a decrepit old man?"

I knew Rudy well enough to know there were still many areas of his life where his competencies were undiminished. But I also knew that now was not the time to point those out to him. Rudy had to find his own way to a new definition of power.

Indeed, there can be a different definition of power, one that is not gender specific and one that is not affected when illness, injury, or diminishing sexual potency come into play. There are two aspects to this new kind of power—the *power to be* and the *power to love and be loved*. The power to be means to appreciate the gift of simply being alive. Actually, every one of us has this power from the time we are born. Men and women possess it equally. The conventional notion of power implies power *over* something or someone; it is hierarchical. That kind of power is something we can lose; competing with others to maintain it as you age is a fool's game that will never outrun the race of aging.

Aiden put it this way: "When I was young, I was small for my age and teased for it. Fortunately, I had the brains and education to find meaning and satisfaction in literature. Now my health has gone south, again. I feel lucky because I have the know-how to make the best out of the life I have. It's not exactly the lemons into lemonade thing, more like finding joy wherever I can. Nothing lasts forever."

The power to love and be loved is similar to the power to be, but it is relational. It has to do with our intimate connection with others. In my own example, there was never a time when I felt closer to my wife, Amy, or loved her more, than when I lay helpless in the hospital. She was there for me every moment of the day, and, undistracted by my ordinary activities and ways of being in the world, I could simply bask in her unconditional regard and return it to her.

I once interviewed a psychologist who has been leading a men's group for twenty-five years. When I asked him what was the most important insight he had gleaned from observing men over such a long time, he replied, "For each of them the need for connection is uppermost. They come to the group with a variety of ostensible reasons, but all of them, I think, were searching for connection. Some of them took years before they could open up and share their vulnerability with the group."

Connection is, indeed, a different kind of power, a kind that, once established, never leaves us.

Vulnerability

Connection also means vulnerability. The following true story illustrates this. Duane's wife was critically ill, and she had been in the hospital for several weeks following complications from surgery. She was not getting better. In fact, each day she got a little weaker, and the doctors were not optimistic. "We're doing our best," her surgeon said, "but I'm sorry to have to tell you that she may not survive."

Duane was distraught. In the midst of this crisis he made an appointment with Rev. Hanson, the hospital's in-house chaplain. As soon as Duane sat down with the chaplain, he began to cry. "I don't know what to do," he said. "I feel totally helpless. I'm powerless; I'm weak. I can't do anything for my wife, and she is just fading away, every day more and more."

Rev. Hanson listened patiently and didn't say anything. After a while Duane stopped talking and just sat slumped in his chair.

"This vulnerability you are feeling," Rev. Hanson said quietly. "That is not weakness. That is strength. You are feeling helpless because you love your wife. Your vulnerability is coming from love, and it is not weakness, but strength. Whatever happens, that kind of strength is what will get you through this."

As it happened, after a few more days Duane's wife turned a corner and began to slowly improve. Eventually she made a full recovery.

Rev. Hanson counseled men like Duane every day. He knew from his training and long experience that men in Duane's situation exacerbate their suffering by mistaking their vulnerability for weakness. Their tears are not weakness, but strength.

"Suck it up," boys of Duane's generation were told. But under the duress of a critical situation such as Duane's, that hard shell of sucking it up will crack. And once it cracks, and the false shell of strength and power is gone, there is a chance that the true power of real connection and vulnerability can shine through.

Although aging does involve the gradual loss of virility, power, and control, this loss has its positive aspects. Aging men can learn, just as Duane did, that vulnerability and weakness offer their own form of power, and that true power does not come from without, but from within. What's more, power is not the only signifier of male identity; there are others that can provide support and nourishment up to the very end of life.

Deep Mind Reflections

There are two deep mind reflections for this chapter: one emphasizing power, and the other focused on vulnerability. The first one, on power, is designed to help you discover how much your identity is connected to the powers you think you have. Do you think you would still be the same person without those powers?

Let's find out. Begin as usual by sitting quietly for a while and calming your mind, letting your thoughts settle and focusing your attention on your physical awareness—where you are sitting, where your body is in the room, how your body feels, and what kind of mood you are in.

Next, bring up the keyword *power*. Repeat it a few times silently to yourself—*power, power. Power* is one of those words that packs a real punch. Just saying the word *power* evokes anticipation of using that power for some purpose.

When you have the word *power* solidly in focus, search for an image to go with it. You may need to cycle through several pictures in your mind before you settle on something that represents not just power generally, but *your* power. So, for example, you may first come up with electrical power, nuclear power, financial power, political power, and so on. But these are abstract uses of power and not personal to you. You may want to use the adjective *powerful* as it pertains to you. What picture or image evokes for you a sense of being personally powerful in some way? If you manage people at work, for example, you have a kind of personal power over them. You could picture yourself sitting at your desk or at the head of a table during a staff meeting.

If you are physically large or strong, that also represents personal power. You might have athletic accomplishments from when you were young that you could bring to mind. If you work out or lift weights, that is an exercise of power too. I have one friend who told me that whenever he is disappointed or angry about something, he goes to the gym and "takes it out on the weight machines." In other words, he restores his internal sense of power by flexing his muscles.

The image that comes to mind for me is the online FreeCell solitaire game that I often play on my smartphone to relax my mind. I compete with myself to see how fast I can solve it. I notice how I feel when I solve it quickly: Powerful! Fast! Smart! I can palpably feel the lift in my mood as I make the last move and the game tells me I have won.

See if you can find an image from your life that gives you that lift.

Rest with your keyword and key image for a while, and watch how evoking power in this way makes you feel. Is it a good feeling?

Most men would probably say so. Power is our touchstone. We are probably hard-wired for it; genetically, we are primates, after all. When chimpanzees or gorillas see a predator approaching, the males form a circle around the females and children and prepare to protect the group by rearing up and making themselves appear large—manifesting power.

Before you allow this first reflection on power to dissipate, reflect on the fact that, in so many ways, aging means a decrease in power. It is true that some forms of power—wealth, for example—can increase with age, which may be why many men work so hard late into middle age to grow more wealth even though they already have more than enough. But most kinds of power decrease with each passing year. It is not easy to face this fact head-on, which is why I see the task of facing aging as having a heroic aspect. It takes courage.

The second deep mind reflection complements the first; it focuses on vulnerability or weakness. Earlier in this chapter I told the story of Duane, whose wife was critically ill, and Rev. Hanson, the chaplain he consulted. Rev. Hanson worked to reframe Duane's seeming weakness as strength. This reflection will follow this same trajectory. Your keyword could be *vulnerability*, though that is rather long to say or think. The word *weakness* is simpler. You can say it silently to yourself: *Weakness, weakness* or *weak, weak. Weak* has several flavors of meaning. It could mean physically weak, as when you are ill. It could mean psychologically weak—for example, when you know you should apologize to a good friend for a rude comment but are too embarrassed to do it. It could mean morally or ethically weak, as when you find some money lying on the street and know you should try to find its owner, but pocket it instead.

The word *weakness* typically carries a sense of self-criticism or negative judgment, for example, in the phrase, "How could I have been so weak?" But weakness needn't be a criticism; it could just be a neutral fact. As you linger on the word, see if you can reverse or neutralize that negativity and instead feel that neutrality. "Yes, sometimes I'm weak, but that's okay, that's just how it is sometimes. I can't always be strong."

As for a key image, try drawing on your life experience for various situations in which you might have felt weak. It could be a time when you were ill or a time when you felt frightened or apprehensive.

Try doing the same for your key image. When I try this, I immediately picture myself lying flat on my back in the rehab hospital. I remember how weak I felt then, but now, with the passage of time, I can see it more neutrally. That's just how it was: I was very ill, and that is why I was weak. There was no fault or blame.

Whatever image bubbles up, try to reframe it as Rev. Hanson did for Duane. Vulnerability can be strength; weakness can be a new place from which to become strong. Regardless, weakness need not make you any less valuable or admirable as a person. Weakness recurs regularly in the cycle of life. You have been weak before, and you will be weak again—more frequently, in fact, as you age.

Whether you are weak or strong, you are incontrovertibly *you*. The people who loved you before when you thought of yourself as strong will still love you when you think of yourself as weak. There is no shame in it. Regrettably, in our consumerist, youth-centric culture older people are often perceived as less valuable, less useful—yes, and weaker. There is a new meme circulating recently, one spoken by the young to the old: "Okay, boomer." It's dismissive; it means we older ones don't matter anymore or are out of touch with what is really happening. I can remember when my generation was young; we had a dismissive phrase too: "Don't trust anyone over thirty." These are ageist put-downs. Ageism in the workplace and in society at large, arising with each generation, is regrettable and corrosive. We cannot control these social trends; they are part of the dark underbelly of social attitudes. But you can control how you feel about yourself.

The life you have lived, the contributions you have made—as well as the people you have loved and who have loved you—are your authentic, inviolate story. Rest easy with that, and the various declines that come with aging will not be so hard.

There is a movement—especially among the uber-wealthy barons of high-tech—to push back aging, to defeat aging, to live forever, to upload your brain into a computer, and so on. Some of these highly successful people—who have never seen a problem they couldn't solve—seem quite convinced that immortality is right around the corner and that they will be the ones to bring it to you.

Don't be deceived. It won't happen. Don't pay a fortune to have your body preserved in a cryogenic chamber to await a future time when your terminal disease can be cured and you can be revived. (Yes, there are actually companies that market this possibility). Life comes from the gift of being born, and death is simply the natural outcome of that life.

When I was thirty-five and had cancer, well-meaning people would ask, "Do they know why you got it?" Somehow, it seemed to them, if I could tell them a cause it would assuage their own discomfort and anxiety about my illness. I would always give them the Buddhist answer, "Because I have a body." For that is what Buddhism teaches: sickness and old age are simply outcomes of being born, of having a body.

So it is not a mystery why our body finally breaks down and dies; it is, if anything, the natural outcome of a blessing. The real mystery is what miracle allows the body to function flawlessly for as many years as it does. If I ask myself, "Why am I weak?" the best answer might be, "Because I am alive."

4

THE MASCULINE STEREOTYPE

We live in a time when gender roles are becoming more fluid and gender categories are being reimagined, but readers fifty and older will have grown up when these roles and categories were more narrowly and rigidly defined. Back in the 1950s and 1960s, men could answer the question "What does it mean to be a man?" by referring to these conventional stereotypes, which were upheld by a vocabulary of catch phrases such as "Don't be a wimp." Society provided norms and definitions of maleness that were pushed onto most men and growing boys whether they were true or not and whether they fit or not. The unfortunate reality is that the masculine stereotype of those days excluded or marginalized whole categories of people that only recently have come to be recognized and respected. The current term LGBTQ—which stands for "lesbian, gay, bisexual, transgender, queer"—defines and legitimizes some of these marginalized categories. It is an effort to create a new vocabulary to include categories of people that the old masculine stereotype previously blotted out.

The masculine stereotype of fifty years ago was an unwritten code of language and behavior—sometimes referred to as the *boy code*. Back then it was common for parents to tell their sons, "Grow a thick skin." In those days it was a social norm that boys and men didn't express emotions openly—especially sadness, fear, or anxiety. When I was growing up, I often heard the phrase, "Suck it up, kid." And the worst thing you could call another boy was "sissy" or "fag."

A respondent on my aging blog remembers these taunts:

"Losers don't make excuses."

"Are you going to whine or win?"

"Nice guys finish last."

These phrases had real power and were part of bullying. Through painful insults, they formed our identities as we grew up.

These schoolyard taunts are all crude expressions of a certain set of ideas—deeply held and enforced by the surrounding culture—of what it means to be a boy or man. These ideas hold that men are strong, not weak. They don't show vulnerability. They are winners, not losers. They can accept and endure pain without complaining. This masculine stereotype is not limited to America. It can be found the world over. For example, one African tribe initiates their young men into adulthood in a painful ceremony. The young men have to crawl—mostly naked—through stinging nettles. They are also beaten in particularly painful places, such as on the bony part of their ankle. In some cases, mud is allowed to dry into a mask on their face, which will reveal a telltale crack if an initiate flinches or winces. If he does, the young man is labeled a coward.[1]

It is also worth remembering that while only a fraction of today's young men serve in the military, when today's aging men were boys, most of their fathers had served in either World War II or the Korean War, and the military culture of those wars upheld the masculine stereotype of courage, stoicism, willingness to face injury and death, and obedience to masculine authority. When I was in elementary school, my best friend's father was a Marine veteran of Iwo Jima. This father

EVERY BREATH, NEW CHANCES

still had his Marine helmet and equipment belt, and my friend and I used to "play war" with these relics with a sense that war and the masculine values that went with it were an ordinary part of everyone's life.

This masculine stereotype, we must add, is largely a heterosexual standard. Gay men have a different internal experience of strength, emotion, and character, and as boys must endure these taunts as an aggressive form of bullying. Gay and transgender teen boys have rates of depression and suicide many times greater than hetero and cis boys, partly because of this bullying.

Regarding men's reluctance to express emotions: although it is not really true that strong men don't cry, there is some scientific basis for male emotional reticence. Today's understanding of brain physiology—documented in books such as Louann Brizendine's *The Female Brain* and *The Male Brain*—confirms that men and women experience and express their emotions in different ways and at different speeds. This is significant, since aging issues are not primarily intellectual, but emotional.[2]

When I talk to men about aging, they are quite ready to acknowledge the intellectual facts and figures of aging; they can talk about gaining weight, drinking too much, having more physical ailments and injuries. But the emotional facets of aging—the anxious sense of gradual loss and the diminution of future possibilities and accomplishment—are harder for them to access. In my interviews, I often hear the masculine stereotype being expressed and echoed as settled fact.

"Being a man means stepping up," Charles said to me when I asked him what he thought it meant to be a man. "Doing what you have to do."

"Being in control," said Peter, answering the same question. "Not messing around."

"Taking charge," said Richard. "Men take charge. That's what we do."

We see this stereotype frequently in popular entertainment too. In *The Godfather*, Vito Corleone says to his son Michael, "I spend my life trying not to be careless. Women and children can be careless, but not men."

So it used to be and often still is. Men are strong, not weak; they suppress emotion; they don't show vulnerability; they don't make mistakes. These attitudes still are common and deeply embedded—regrettably so, since they do not serve men well, particularly in the context of aging. A man can't beat aging by trying to be a tough guy. Aging will always win that battle. It might seem for a while that aging can be tackled by putting your dukes up, but then aging throws a roundhouse punch—a bum knee, a troubling diagnosis, a sudden illness, financial reverses, any number of troubles that no tough guy act can solve.

Emotions

There is a difference between a thought and an emotion—a difference that many men fail to recognize or acknowledge. Thoughts express concepts and judgments, while emotions express feelings. They are entirely different experiences. A thought is mental; its world is the brain. But while an emotion has a mental component, it is also physical—its world is the body. When you are angry, your whole body is transformed. Your face flushes, your heart beats faster, the muscles in your neck tense, and your tone of voice changes. Those things don't typically happen with a mere thought, unless it's a thought that accompanies an emotion.

Ted spoke up in a workshop about a recent visit to his doctor, who told him he needed to cut down on his drinking and lose weight.

"How did you feel about that?" I asked.

"I felt criticized," Ted replied.

Ted said he *felt* criticized, but in actuality the word *criticized* refers to a thought, not an emotion. It was Ted's intellectual characterization of the doctor's comment. Whatever emotion he felt was something quite different. I had no doubt that Ted felt an emotion, but he didn't acknowledge it or say what it was. I could have suggested to Ted some actual emotions to choose from—anger, sadness, or fear, perhaps—but I'm not sure he would have understood the value of selecting one over the other.

There is one emotion that men are inclined to express openly: anger. That is an emotion that the masculine stereotype allows; anger expresses aggression and shows that you are a "real" man. The columnist George Will, writing about anger in an August 2019 piece, said, "James Q. Wilson, the most accomplished social scientist of his time, noted that genetics and neuroscience suggest that self-control is more attenuated in men than in women. The part of the brain that stimulates anger and aggression is larger in men, and the part that restrains anger is smaller in men."[3]

Anger, as a genuine emotion, is most commonly employed as an aggressive response—although it sometimes functions simply to let a man know that something within him needs attention. At the opposite end of the emotional spectrum from anger is crying. Crying is tender, not hard; vulnerable, not aggressive; exposed, not hidden. Men are generally uncomfortable when tears come, especially in front of others. For them, crying is a troubling loss of control, and if others see it, they can feel embarrassed and humiliated. If they feel tears coming on, men will leave the room and tend to their tears in private—"pulling themselves together"—before returning to the group.

Men may feel bewildered and disoriented by tears and may not know why they are crying or what they are feeling. One psychologist I know uses what he calls a "feeling wheel"—a circular chart with the names of various emotions on it—to help his male clients who are crying identify a genuine emotion that best reflects their actual emotional state.

It is a common misunderstanding to think that an emotion comes first and its bodily sensations—lump in the throat, tightness in the chest—follow. Current research shows that the opposite is true: the physical sensation comes first, and the felt emotion follows.[4] The key to properly identifying an emotion is to focus clearly on the physical sensations you have in your body.

When Ted felt criticized by his doctor telling him he needed to cut down on his drinking, he might have tuned in to his bodily sensations and realized that he was angry.

"Yes, I was pissed," I finally got him to say when I asked him to remember how his body felt in that moment. "I don't like people telling me what to do."

Be aware that the older you get, the more you may find people (like a doctor or a financial planner) telling you what to do. This is one aspect of the loss of independence that is part of aging, and it happens first in subtle, then not-so-subtle ways.

Gender Roles and Aging

Masculinity is a social role, not necessarily the fixed biological condition it was assumed to be until recently. Today we know that gender is different from sex; while *sex* refers to certain genetic traits assigned at birth, *gender* is understood by many researchers to be influenced by a range of societal, environmental, and genetic factors.[5] Gender appears to be a complex characteristic deeply embedded in the psyche of an individual. For example, someone born in a woman's body may identify deeply as a man—in other words, he is a transgender man. It is also important to differentiate gender from sexual orientation. Gay men are sexually attracted to other men, but they have a continuum of attitudes and expression regarding masculinity itself. Some gay men see themselves—and may be perceived by others—as hewing to the masculine stereotype of strength, courage, toughness, and stoicism. There are pro football players who have come out as gay, for example. Other gay men express a persona more commonly associated with a feminine stereotype—emotional sensitivity, artistic proclivity, gentleness, and nurturing. And these expressions are not necessarily mutually exclusive. How a man experiences his own aging depends to a large extent on the social role and gender characteristics he has been raised in and accustomed to.

That being said, aging is only partly personal; some aspects of aging are universal. While each person will have his own unique experience of aging, there is also the shared experience of aging that everyone has. At the personal level, how a man ages will be colored by the gender role and gender qualities he possesses. At the universal level, aging is independent of gender. The slow decline of youthful vigor and physical abilities, the onset of various chronic and acute illnesses, the closing off of life possibilities, livelihoods, and careers, as well as the new chances that open up as aging proceeds, are universal qualities of being alive. In fact, we could say that aging happens because birth has happened; aging is the natural unfolding of the gift of life.

Identity: Who Am I Really?

There are at least three aspects to being a man: biology, gender, and sexual orientation. In addition, there is what we could call *core identity, soul,* or *innermost self,* which is apart from these. Your core identity is beyond roles and categories; it is the pure living being that came into this world when you were born and will leave this world when you die. It is also the part of you that doesn't age in an ordinary sense. Of course, in most respects you are a completely different person than you were when you were five, ten, or twenty years old. But there is a part of you that is continuous with who you were at those younger ages. This is what I mean by core identity.

It is vital to include core identity in any comprehensive discussion of aging, because your core identity is not just male, female, or any gender type along the spectrum. Your core identity carries the essence of your simply being alive.

There is a story from the Buddhist tradition that wonderfully illustrates this point, besides being preternaturally modern in its perspective. The story concerns a Buddhist monk named Shariputra, a celibate male monastic who lived in ancient India and who believed that women were inferior to men in all things—a view that was normative for his time and culture. According to the story, while Shariputra was at a monastic gathering he was confronted by a goddess who challenged his religious understanding.

"I possess all the wisdom of the gods," the goddess said to Shariputra. "Your monkish ideas are elementary compared to mine."

"That cannot be," Shariputra replied. "In our monastic community, we are taught that the most senior woman is junior to the most junior man. We are also taught that the best way for a woman to achieve wisdom is to be reborn as a man. I look forward to your rebirth as a man so you can achieve full enlightenment, which requires the body of a man to attain."

"I am also gifted with great magical powers," the goddess said. She then snapped her fingers and instantly Shariputra's body became her body, while the goddess's body became that of Shariputra.

Shariputra was shocked beyond belief. He looked down at his female body clothed in the goddess's clothing and trembled with fear.

"What do you think, Shariputra?" the goddess laughed. "Are you any less wise than you were just a moment before, now that you have taken my body as your own?"

"I don't know what to think," Shariputra stammered. "I think I am the same, but I am clearly not the same. How did you do that? What does this mean?"

The goddess snapped her fingers again, and she and Shariputra both resumed their original forms. "Shariputra," the goddess said, "the essence of a person does not depend on their outward form as man or woman. The essence of a person is beyond all such limitations. This is my teaching for you."

Shariputra, relieved to have his old body back, bowed in acknowledgment of the goddess's superior understanding.

This story is recorded in a Buddhist scripture entitled *Vimalakirti Sutra*. The societies of India in the fifth century BCE, like many ancient societies and even many contemporary ones, were patriarchal, male dominated, and suffused with a firm belief in male superiority; these attitudes are reflected in the story about Shariputra.

The story of Shariputra makes two important points about gender and identity. First, men have deeply held attitudes about who they are as men. Shariputra is one example of that. Second, we are not defined solely by our physical body, our biology, or our perceived gender. There is a part of us—the deepest and most important part—that is beyond all of that, as the goddess taught. This deepest part is our core identity, and core identity stands above and apart from all the ideas and feelings we have about aging. As one of my Buddhist teachers often said, "The most important fact is that you actually exist right now in this present moment. Remember this truth, and you will have the strength to face any adversity."

To put it another way, fundamentally, our existence is not defined by being a man or a woman, gay or straight, or cisgender, transgender, or nonbinary, but simply by the fact of our being here at all—the gift of life that continues until our last moment.

Deep Mind Reflection: Being a Man

The purpose of this reflection is to help you explore what you think being a man is. You may not have thought about it in so many words, but if you are like most men, you hold deep core beliefs about being a man. To begin exploring this, you could start with that actual phrase—*being a man*—as your keyword. *Being a man, being a man*—what feelings and images come up for you when you silently repeat that phrase? It is worth spending some time trying out various mental pictures of what you think being a man is.

One approach would be to visualize a man whom you have looked up to in your life—your father, grandfather, or uncle perhaps, or a teacher, mentor, or trusted friend. This approach draws on the fact that your sense of yourself as a man was probably influenced by the men you grew up with and looked up to when you were younger. They were your models. As you continue your reflection and your search for an appropriate key image, you need to understand that the attitudes we have about being a man lie fairly deep in our psyche. They are not qualities that you typically think much about; rather, they are simply part of the substructure that holds together who you think you are. Repeating your key phrase and trying on your key image will help you bring this substructure into view.

If you are using as a key image an older male relative who is still living, that image may include that person's age. Picturing an aging father or grandfather evokes the image of your future self. Don't be surprised if your key image turns into an image of yourself as you might be at that age.

Because "being a man" is such a loaded expression, at first you might try just working with this key phrase by itself, without a key image, just to see what associations this phrase brings up. You might find that your deep mind finds various ways to complete a sentence beginning "Being a man means ..."

Some of my interviewees tried this approach. Here are some possibilities that they brought up.

"Being a man means being strong."

"Being a man means being responsible."

"Being a man means not backing down."

"Being a man means making a living and supporting a family."

Another approach would be to concentrate just on your key image, and see where that leads you. Images are the natural language of deep mind, and they also tend to be more emotional. So, for example, focusing on an image of your grandfather will bring with it the emotional connection you had with your grandfather, as well as the memories of the activities you did together—fishing, perhaps, or woodworking or going to the movies. See where this initial image leads you. The image of your grandfather could morph into the image of another older male friend or relative, bringing up different memories of feelings and activities that connected you to their example of being a man.

Deep Mind Reflection: Core Identity

Reflection into core identity takes you in a different direction. Core identity is outside of gender, beyond male and female; it is who you are *aside* from being a man. You could formulate your key phrase to express that in just those words: *Who am I outside of being a man?* After a few repetitions of this phrase you could shorten it: *Who am I?* or *Who am I really?*

One obvious answer that may come to you is your name. For me that would be, "I am Lewis Richmond." Yes, that is indeed my name, but is that who I am really? My name is what I call myself and what I am called by others, but I could change my name, and I would still be me. My name is not who I am really.

Another answer that might come to mind is your occupation. I could say about myself, "I am a writer." Being a writer may be what I do for a living, but there is a lot more to who I am than my occupation. Besides, I may not always be a writer. Remember Len, the teacher who was forced to take early retirement and was furious about it? If he were doing this reflection, the phrase "I am a teacher" would undoubtedly bring up feelings of anger and sadness. Yes, Len used to work as a teacher, he has the skills of a teacher and could find another teaching job, but at the moment he spoke up, he was not actively a teacher.

So who was he really? Len might be someone who could really benefit from a reflection on his core identity. Part of his anger stemmed from his strong identification with his being a teacher and his loss of that identity. Even though he lost his job as a teacher, his core identity was not touched. Realizing that could be the first step in his building a new life and career.

The key image that accompanies your investigation of core identity might not be obvious immediately. Core identity is actually something of a mystery, an aspect of yourself buried deep in the heart of who you are. Rather than trying too hard to imagine a key image that fits, just choose the first image that occurs to you. For example, you could picture the photograph on your driver's license. We already know that that picture does not represent your core identity, but it is connected to some aspect of your identity. Start there and see where that tentative identity leads when you follow it more deeply.

For myself, when I bring that photo to mind and let myself freely associate, I start to remember other photos of myself at various ages—one when I was a baby, one when I was eight years old, and so on. I then realize that while the person in each of those photos looks different, the core identity in the soul of each one is the same.

As a final reflection, you could ask yourself, *How old is this core identity of mine?* Is it your birthday age, your biological age (the age you feel physically), your mental age, or some other age entirely? Don't be surprised if you have trouble coming up with an answer to this question. You may discover that there is an aspect of core identity that lives apart from all of those other ages—that is, in effect, ageless. Knowing and touching a part of yourself that is ageless is a wonderful counterpoint to all your other aging issues and difficulties.

In asking all these questions and pondering your answers, you are trusting your deep mind to communicate to you a well-earned wisdom, one that you have spent a lifetime nourishing and that is now available to nourish you. That is a lot to ponder. You might want to delve into these deep mind reflections several times over days or weeks. I can't predict what you will discover; everyone is different. But I would guess that at the end of this process you will know more about who you are not just as a man, or even as an aging man, but also as a unique, precious living being who is beyond all thoughts or limitations of being a man.

These truths are vital for your progress on the aging journey. You may not know exactly where you are headed; that is not known. But at least you will better understand who it is that is making the journey. That, in the end, may be more important.

5

THE DECADES OF AGING

The process of aging is not a smooth, continuous trajectory from youth to old age. It happens—or feels as though it happens—in distinct, identifiable stages. We often identify these stages through significant life events—the last child leaving home, a divorce, a second marriage, retirement—but colloquially we tend to think of aging's stages in decades: our fifties, sixties, seventies, eighties, and beyond. A birthday with a zero—"Oh my God, I'm sixty!"—is a major, sometimes bittersweet, signpost. This chapter can be thought of as a roadmap of the decades, with markers to help you locate yourself on the map. Each decade has characteristics common to most people in them. Men in their fifties, for example, though still near the height of their earning power, are beginning to notice that their physical strength and endurance are not what they once were—particularly if they have an athletic background and are accustomed to ease in their physical activity.

To help us explore these decades, I'll use the schema of Erikson's eight life stages that we discussed in chapter 1. Though Erikson's stages begin with infancy and continue into old age, as we discussed earlier, his last two stages are the ones relevant to aging—*generativity* and *deep acceptance*. Generativity—spanning roughly the ages from thirty to sixty-five—is a time of mature adulthood when a man contributes to society through children and family, career and livelihood. Deep acceptance typically begins around age sixty-five, when a man starts to look back on his life and begins to assess how his life has unfolded and what he has done.

This shift from generativity to deep acceptance is not always easy to recognize. My friend Stan was sixty-five when my book *Aging as a Spiritual Practice* was published. I gave him a copy, but he told me he didn't want to read it. "I'll read it when I'm old," he said. "Eighty or so." Two years later Stan died of a fast-growing cancer. He and his wife were completely unprepared. Cancer, they had thought, was something that happened when you were old. Stan hadn't realized that, in terms of susceptibility to illness, he was already old.

Health care providers I have talked to tell me that men and women seem to become aware of aging at different speeds. Beginning in their mid- to late fifties, women deal with "empty nest" syndrome and a feeling of becoming invisible, while men of that age are (or think they are) still powerful, still attractive, still strong and vital. For the next twenty years or so, men lag behind women in aging awareness, until, in their seventies, these differences even out. This lag time becomes important as men traverse the decades of aging.

As you read this chapter, you may be tempted to skip ahead to the decade you are in (or to skip decades you're not in yet). I encourage to read about all the decades. For example, if you are in your fifties, you may find it edifying to learn about the decades ahead of you and what gifts and challenges they will bring. Or, if you are in your seventies or eighties, looking back to an earlier period of your life may be useful in coming to terms with the age you are now.

Until recently it was less common for a man to live past his seventies. In 1950 average life expectancy for men was around sixty-five.

Now that life expectancy is nearly eighty, and some men—think of ex-presidents George H. W. Bush and Jimmy Carter—live productive, meaningful lives well into their nineties.

The Starting-to-Age Fifties

Many men do not think much about aging when they are in their fifties, unless they have been hit with a serious injury or illness. The fifties are the crest of the curve, so to speak—or so it would seem for those in the professional class: lawyers, doctors, educators, business managers, and executives. For men who work with their bodies or hands—tradesmen, craftspeople, athletes, builders, and factory workers who fabricate things and work with materials—the fifties are a time when injuries or chronic physical conditions often become a real problem and a livelihood threat. The carpenter who remodeled our house—someone who could easily lift a hundred-pound sack of concrete—recounted to me a whole litany of injuries, beginning with his youthful days as a minor league baseball pitcher.

"I got nothing left in my right shoulder, no cartilage or anything," he told me one day. "Rotator cuff."

"That must hurt," I observed.

"I always hurt," he said.

If men in their fifties have children, these children are probably in high school or college. Raising children to adulthood and mentoring them so they can succeed as adults, is the classic task of generativity. If a man does not have a family, there are still many ways he can express generativity—in career, in creative contribution to society, in philanthropy, coaching, teaching, and volunteer work. Generativity, according to Erikson, is an archetypal need to be a productive and important member of society. Every person feels it, and every society recognizes it—whether traditional, modern, or postmodern.

In my fifties I was a professional with rising prospects in two fields: software and writing. My software company was expanding, I had six employees, and I expected soon to have more. The prospect of rapid growth of my company leading to an acquisition was not an unrealistic fantasy. Cashing out in software sometimes happened in those heady days, though as it turned out it did not happen to me. I was working on my first book, *Work as a Spiritual Practice*. I also had a nine-year-old son. I was well positioned to express my generativity in a variety of satisfying ways. My bout with encephalitis brought all of that to a screeching halt, but until then I was riding high.

Taking my experience as typical, we might label the decade of the fifties as the decade of possible dreams. In that sense, this decade marks the summit of ambition and an expansionist vision that peaks just at the point that lamp of the physical body—and probably the career reality—is starting to dim. In our fifties, aging—like it or not—has begun.

My experience of family in my fifth decade is typical of a married professional man. Straight men in their fifties who are single or divorced have the additional advantage of still being able to attract women their own age or younger. As Henry Kissinger once said, "Power is the great aphrodisiac."

However, gay men in their fifties may have a different experience. They can't compete as well with younger men in physical attractiveness. If an older gay man is not already married or in a committed relationship, he may find himself lonely, even if he has money and a successful career.

I was speaking with Jay, a golf pro at a country club. Jay had just turned fifty-six and was telling me how it felt to be his age. Jay had gone through a divorce a few years back and was currently single.

"I feel great," Jay said. "I'm still in great shape physically. I work out three or four times a week; I still play eighteen holes a couple times a week when I am not working. Usually I shoot a couple under par. I'm not living with a woman now but I have a steady relationship, which is great. All in all, things are good."

"Do you feel like you are starting to age?"

"Not really," Jay replied quickly. "I'm losing my looks just a bit and starting to gray a little around the edges, but I'm out of the singles scene, so it doesn't matter."

"How's your overall health?" I said.

"Couldn't be better," Jay said. "My doc says I have the body of someone half my age." He paused. "I've taken a few hits though. I twisted my knee playing pickup basketball a few months back, and I guess that's a sport I'm going to have to give up. That's okay, though. Golf's my game. I can play golf until I'm eighty."

I didn't want to ask Jay about his divorce, though in previous conversations he'd told me a little about it. As he recounted it, the divorce was amicable mostly because he gave his ex-wife everything she asked for. "It broke her heart, though," he added.

Jay was typical of healthy men in their fifties, still actively engaged in work and career, still thinking of himself as young, attractive, and healthy and not concerned about what the next few years might bring. There is a catch-phrase often heard these days: *sixty is the new forty*. It's true that with better diet, better medicine, and attention to health basics such as weight, diet, alcohol consumption, and exercise, many men enter their fifth decade looking and feeling younger than they did in previous generations. That's a good thing.

But the fifth decade is also a time to lay down good habits for the future regarding health. Any weight a man puts on in his fifties will be harder to lose with each passing year and decade. Jay was off to a good start, but he was a professional athlete and sportsman. He was only one major shoulder or hip injury away from a sudden career crisis.

The Declining-Energy Sixties

The transition from generativity to deep acceptance is gradual. In generativity, a man is still deeply engaged in a busy, fulfilling present and a vision of an imagined future. Deep acceptance starts to occur when that imagined future begins to fade, and a man begins to look more backward than forward, assessing the accomplishments he has made and the work he has done. The sixth decade is when this shift typically begins.

Dan was an example of a man in his early sixties who had not yet begun to look back. He was still completely engaged in his busy career life, which was, to hear him describe it, all encompassing.

Dan had left the corporate life some twenty-five years before to open a restaurant—his lifelong dream. The restaurant was a success, and Dan was doing well.

"Yeah, the restaurant keeps cooking along, so to speak, and I've got a great family. Life is good."

He told me that his two sons were just finishing college and preparing for exciting careers, one in medicine and the other in international relations. "They really turned out well," Dan said. "It's really great to see your kids enter the adult world and prosper."

When I asked him how he felt about aging he said, "No complaints, no major illnesses or health problems. Had to have my shoulder fixed up, but I had a great surgeon, he says I'll be back to go in no time. I'm really enjoying being older; everything is breaking my way."

"Have you thought about how things might look in another five or ten years?" I asked.

For the first time in our conversation, Dan hesitated. "I really haven't," he said after a while. "Of course, we've got our financial plans and retirement all worked out, but I guess I'm enjoying life too much now to really worry about anything that far down the road."

"In ten years you'll be seventy-three," I said.

"Wow," Dan replied. "Yeah, that's right. Seventy-three. That sounds old!" He paused. "Well, I guess I'll deal with it when I get there."

For many men the stars are not so nicely aligned as they were for Dan. Some men are feeling the physical, mental, and emotional effects of aging by the time they reach sixty.

Nathan, a classical musician who toured several months a year, said to me, "In my line of work, it's after you turn sixty that you feel your energy starting to tail off. Each year a little more. I used to be able to get off the plane at noon, be at the hotel by two, take a nap, work out for an hour, shower and dress, and be at the concert hall by six, ready to tear into a two-hour concert with energy to spare. Now I can't do that. A lot of times I arrange to fly in the night before so I can get a good night's sleep and adjust to the jet lag before I'm ready to face the next day. I take care of myself; I have to with my travel schedule. But I'll tell you, the years wear you down. I don't know how long I'll be able to keep this up."

Nathan's travel-intensive career meant that for him the energy decline of the sixth decade was quite noticeable. But it's true for all of us. Each living species has its maximum lifespan. For a fruit fly it might be a few weeks. For a fox or opossum, it is around two years. With enough to eat, clean water, and good medical care, people are now living to be eighty, ninety, and beyond. Then there are those titans of the high-tech industry who aspire to lengthen this lifespan using various methods—a calorie-restricted diet, exotic supplements and vitamins, cold showers, even low-level radiation to the brain. There is now serious discussion of uploading your brain into a computer and keeping your mind alive indefinitely.

Looking beneath the surface of these science fiction pronouncements, I sense a shadow there. Most of these long-life proponents are young, wealthy, highly successful men. Everything they have touched has turned to gold; why not life itself? Science has already nearly doubled the average lifespan, from forty-nine years in 1900 to eighty years today. But the fear of growing old is different from growing old itself. That fear, like any fear, is an unwelcome guest. We do not want it. We want a drug, a medicine, an elixir, a potion, a new technology to vanquish it. But this fear is not fleeting or fragmentary. It is part of the fabric of life itself. We can't have our life without the fear. They go together.

My sixth decade was different from most. I was still recovering from my brain infection and brush with death. When I was critically ill, I had thought I would die, or that I would be permanently disabled, or that I would lose my livelihood, my home, my property and possessions—everything! I had been, in the words of one of my therapists, to the "mountaintop of worry" and was slowly coming down from it. Eventually I realized that none of those dire consequences would come true. Eventually I got my life back.

But it was a long journey down from that mountaintop.

The Seventies: Impermanence and Chaos

I am seventy-two, so I can write about the seventh decade from personal experience. I remember, when I was sixty-nine, asking my wife, who is a couple years older than I, what it's like to turn seventy. "It will be fine," she assured me. "You'll still feel the same."

I wasn't so sure. Somehow being in my sixties still seemed young-ish to me. The mind plays tricks with aging numbers. When you are in your sixties, you think, "I'm not really so old, plenty of future left." But as the door to the seventies opens, you think, "Well, the sixties turned out okay, I still have game. But seventy! Things are starting to feel shaky. I don't know what's going to happen. A good friend my age had a heart attack last week."

I did my best to set these speculations aside, and see matters through the lens of Buddhist teaching. I realized that what I was really feeling was the quickening drumbeat of what Buddhists call *impermanence*—the realization that no human life is going to last; everything is going to go. For seventy years, I thought, I've cheated the grim reaper, but with each passing month and year, the odds are turning more and more against me. Now I'm becoming a living embodiment of the truth of impermanence.

For much of my early adulthood, I was an active participant in a Buddhist community, where meditation practices and teachings once the exclusive preserve of monks in Asian countries were taken up by ordinary Americans. This "Western Buddhism" had many branches. Some people studied Buddhist texts in their original languages in universities and translated and published many previously unavailable scriptures and commentaries. Buddhist teachers from Asian countries—China, Japan, Korea, Tibet, Burma, and Thailand—came to Western countries to answer the call of seekers of Buddhist wisdom. Religious organizations, retreat centers, and monasteries cropped up everywhere.

I was one of those seekers, and I devoted a good deal of my time to the study of Buddhist teachings and the practice of Buddhist meditation. One of the key Buddhist concepts that I learned and then taught was this idea of impermanence—the realization that everything changes, that nothing lasts, and in the end everything we know and love, including our precious selves, will grow old, weaken, and pass away.

Recently I have come to feel that this term *impermanence* is overly abstract and lacking emotional pungency. It was coined by early translators of Buddhist texts, who were aiming for linguistic accuracy. The actual *feeling* of impermanence isn't abstract at all. It is deeply emotional and sometimes a bit scary.

I'm not sure what word best captures the emotional resonance of impermanence, but *chaos* comes close—*chaos* or *unpredictability*. We all want predictability; we want what happens tomorrow to be a lot like what happened today. We want the people we love to still be there for us, we want our job to be there for us and not vanish in a puff of smoke. We want the weather to be more or less fine. We want everything to run like clockwork, just like the sun that always rises in the East and sets in the West. Most of the time, daily life seems to go that way, but that predictability is actually an illusion. What is really going on is something far more unsettling—the rumbling undercurrent of confusion or chaos.

Every so often this chaos bursts through. We are in a car accident. Someone we love breaks a leg or is hospitalized with a serious illness. The company we work for suddenly goes under, and our secure job is gone. Aging is yet another form of this chaos. At first it doesn't seem so. Yes, we are getting older. We joke about it with our friends. Yet one day we look in the mirror and in a strong light suddenly see how flaccid and wrinkly our once smooth face has become. We go to the doctor for our annual physical. Once it was a boring necessity; now it is cause for a sleepless night. What will those routine tests suddenly reveal? Will the chaos that churns under the seeming calm of life's surface suddenly jump out at us? Will it be cancer or some other frightful disease?

When my wife and I decided to sell our house and move, we didn't realize at first how much chaos it would bring up. At first the chaos was background noise, but once our belongings were moved to storage, and we were camped out in a motel, that background noise became a loud roar. Then it was all chaos, morning to night. All our reliable routines were upended. I barely knew from one day to the next where my wallet and car keys were. Chaos seizes you, and you are its prisoner.

I taught impermanence for years in the Buddhist classes I led. But it was not until we became intentional vagabonds that I really felt the full vertigo of life's chaos. Intellectually I knew that, like everyone, we were always one small step removed from chaos, but it was only when we were camped out in a motel room that it really hit home. That is what impermanence really means.

One day you too may find that all your predictable routines are upended. You never know when it will happen. Sometimes it happens to other people you know, but it is still too close for comfort. In 2017 wildfires destroyed over two thousand homes not thirty miles from our front door. We had friends who were awakened by flames in the middle of the night and fled in their cars, seconds ahead of the raging fires. That same year, in other parts of the country, large cities were inundated by floods.

When your house burns down—or a flood submerges it—you realize in a flash that you never really had a house you could count on, not the way you thought. We are all just one small step away from that kind of annihilation. Aging has the power to surprise us in the same way.

The seventh decade is often the time when the truth of impermanence—and the impending chaos of life's uncertainties—really emerges. The impermanence teachings of Buddhism are good for a young man to read about, but their deep truth only bursts into full flower when you are old. Now, at seventy-two, I feel like I am living out the lessons that the Buddha once taught, and that I only thought I understood when I was young.

The Eighties: A Time for Gratitude

Eighty! I'm not there yet—eight more years to go—but I have spoken to several men who are in their eighties, and what they all seem to say is, "Okay, I get it. I'm really old now." Another sentiment they express is, "I'm glad to have made it this far; I'm grateful."

Indeed, gratitude makes sense when you are eighty or older. You've already outlived the average lifespan for men, so in a sense, you are living on bonus points. Of course, how happy you feel about that depends on your health. In good health, eighty or older feels like a big win. If your health is not so good, the feeling varies. If you have taken good care of yourself in previous decades, the eighth decade is a time to reap the benefit of that. That being said, genes and family history matter too.

I recently started seeing a new cardiologist and told him about my encephalitis. All my doctors thought I would die, I told him, but I proved them wrong. "None of my doctors seemed to have a good explanation."

"I do," he said. "I think it was because you had good genes and a strong heart."

To credit genes for longevity may be giving short shrift to our own efforts to stay healthy. Some men may conclude that if genes are what matters, then what's the point of taking especially good care of yourself? Maybe it's all up to genes and fate! But it's not either/or. A recent study estimates that genes only account for 25 percent of longevity.[1] The title of the article includes the phrase, "It takes two to tango," meaning genes plus lifestyle. So genes matter, but they are only one of many factors ; a healthy lifestyle matters more.

Harold, a dignified man of eighty-four, was a retired physician who still taught occasional seminars in medical school and still published articles in professional journals. Harold and his wife had recently sold the large home in which they had raised four children and moved into a senior living facility. It was not Harold's choice. He told me, "I'd rather die with my boots on." But his wife had a chronic illness and did not want to be a burden to Harold as they grew older. Their new home had a skilled nursing unit and expert caregivers who could help if and when the time came.

"I've had a wonderful life," Harold said. "Looking back, there's nothing I would change, even the hard things. I had a heart attack when I was sixty, and that could have been the ball game. But I beat it, got my health back, and kept going. I think of myself as the Energizer bunny," he chuckled.

By all accounts, Harold seemed like a man who had entered Erikson's eighth stage of deep acceptance. A person in deep acceptance looks back over his life, as Harold did, and—in spite of the "hard things," in Harold's phrase—calls it good. One form this deep acceptance takes is a pleasant nostalgia—the choice to mostly remember the good times. Nostalgia can be one of life's sweeter enjoyments in old age. It is a kind of reflective optimism, choosing to see the bright side in the rearview mirror.

The less happy corollary of nostalgia is regret. Naturally, we all have regrets, but a man who has arrived at deep acceptance chooses not to dwell on them—that is his optimistic bias. Another approach to a regret is to compensate for it with pleasant nostalgia.

Harold offered me an example of this approach. "I actually never set out to be a doctor," he said. "I wanted to be an artist growing up, and I had real talent. I was even accepted at one of the top art schools. But my father was a doctor, a famous hand surgeon, and his idea of giving me a choice in life was to sit me down and say, 'Harold, I want you to know that you can be anything you want in life. Any kind of doctor. You don't have to be a hand surgeon like me.'" Harold laughed. "My dad thought I would starve as an artist.

"He was probably right," Harold said. "I've had so many opportunities to make my patients' lives better, even saving their life sometimes. I wouldn't go back on my life in medicine for anything."

Deep acceptance doesn't mean painting a Pollyanna-ish gloss over the many ups and downs of a whole life. Harold's story shows how to strike a balance between our disappointments and triumphs. When Harold said, "I've had a wonderful life," he was essentially saying that in spite of his regrets, he was happy to color the bulk of his past with the hue of satisfaction.

The eighth decade is quite often the time when even a healthy aging body begins to falter, and a man has to deal with a litany of chronic or acute afflictions—either his own or another's. I got a call recently from a good friend who had been planning a long trip, but suddenly had to cancel when his wife was diagnosed with a stomach tumor and needed immediate surgery. Men in their eighties live in the shadow of such surprises. These men need to manage the worries that can keep them up at night with a cascade of what-ifs. Some couples in their eighties get ahead of the what-ifs by having frank discussions about what either of them would do in such a situation.

I interviewed one woman who wanted nothing better than to have that talk with her husband, but, she said, "He didn't want to talk about that stuff." She felt stuck, and indeed this is another situation where it takes two to tango—in this case, husband and wife. If you are like her husband and don't want to talk about the tough stuff, think again. Aging takes courage, and this is one more example.

How a man copes with the final illnesses of himself or of loved ones is his last heroic project, his final courageous act. Genes matter, and they determine the core features of who we are, but good character, a mature life outlook, and solid plans can all bend that destiny your way. Deep acceptance includes all of that. It is indeed a path of courage.

Deep Mind Reflection: Your Decade

This chapter's deep mind reflection is tied to the decade you are in. Your keyword or phrase could be, *I am in my fifties* or *I am in my sixties.* After a few repetitions you could shorten this phrase to a single word—for example, *fifties.* Alternatively, you could use your exact age—*I am fifty-four*—and then *fifty-four, fifty-four.*

Your age is just a number, but your deep mind feels it as much more. Your deep mind knows the emotional meaning behind the number—which we are most aware of when we hit the zero birthday—fifty, sixty, seventy. That's when people say, "The big six-oh." *Big* means emotionally big. The fact that we say "big" proves these numbers matter, and our deep mind knows it.

Your key image should be something that emerges out of the emotion arising from focusing on your age. Some men feel great about being the age they are; others, the opposite. Your image should capture how you really feel. It is important not to idealize or exaggerate in either direction. Magazines for seniors often feature on their covers some famous celebrity looking fantastic at the age of sixty, seventy, or beyond. That is idealization. I suppose the magazine's intent is to be encouraging. I'm not sure how encouraging it is to compare yourself to someone who probably spends a fortune to look good.

For the purpose of this reflection, it's not how you look; it's how you feel.

I tried this myself, starting with the phrase, *I'm seventy-two.* I imagined myself looking in the mirror—as we all do every morning—and taking stock. I used that as my starting image. I see that my hair is no longer gray. I can pretend it is gray, but it is actually white—as the man who cuts my hair always tells me when I try to tell him it is still partly gray.

My beard at least isn't white; it's still salt-and-pepper. I focus on that fact in my key image. "Still hanging in there," my deep mind comments.

"Not so bad," was the next phrase it offered.

"Doing okay," came next.

I tried to generate an image from the phrase "Doing okay." I thought of the half-hour walk I take every morning along a wooded creek-side path. Until recently I was nursing a minor back injury, a muscle pull that was slowing me down. But in the last few days I haven't been feeling that, and my pace has quickened. *More like the old days*, I thought.

So that became my image of doing okay. In my imagination, I walk that path at my new quicker pace, remembering my keyword: *seventy-two.*

Seventy-two, seventy-two. Doing okay. Walking strong.

That phrase "walking strong" had suddenly appeared, another comment from my deep mind. I felt buoyed up by that phrase.

Try this reflection yourself and see what you come up with. It may be that your deep mind will take you on a bit of an adventure about the feelings you have and the age you are. Coming from your deep mind, it will probably be close to the unvarnished truth. Truth itself can be a medicine as we get older. Truth, whatever it may be, is yet another form of courage in aging.

6

DIVORCED AND SINGLE MEN

I was married when I was twenty, a month before I graduated from college. I am still married to the same woman after fifty-two years. I don't know what percentage of men are like me, but I'm probably quite an outlier on the bell curve of married men. So I have no experience of being divorced or single as an adult. But many men have. According to the U.S. Census, more than 20 percent of men over fifty are single, that is, not living with a spouse or partner. Many more will be single at some future point. This includes men who have never married as well as those who have been divorced or whose partners have died. This statistic has risen over the years as baby boomers have aged, and it means that many men are facing aging largely alone. This has implications for a man's health and even longevity. According to a Harvard health survey, being married increases a man's lifespan, and being single decreases it—a correlation that is not as true for women.[1]

Why might this be? Remember the psychologist who had led a long-term men's group. When I asked him what he felt was the most important issue for men in the group, he replied, "For each of them, the need for connection is uppermost." Clearly close friendships and relationships are valued by men and are keenly important—not just for the personal satisfaction that they bring, but for health. So divorced and single men face an extra set of challenges as they age.

The binary possibility of being married or single is largely an artifact of modern societies. In traditional societies, there have been and still are other possibilities. Although a man might be married, he could spend his days and sometimes nights in the men's lodge, in close comradeship with other men. In some parts of the world, having more than one wife is still not uncommon.

In ancient Athens, aristocratic men generally spent their evenings away from their wives, attending dinner parties—symposia—with their clique of male friends (and perhaps accompanied by a young male lover or a courtesan). And upper-class men in England spent a good deal of time at their club—a male-only haven and refuge from women and family life.

So the notion of a single man is something of a modern social construct. Among today's younger men, this construct is becoming more fluid. Just as gender roles and identities are no longer simply binary, the terms *single* or *married* do not encompass all the varieties of relationships and living situations. The majority of men over fifty, however, more often hew to the old-fashioned binary model of being either married or single. And single older men are prone to loneliness.

Jeremy is a psychologist whose clientele consists entirely of older men. I asked him what is the most common symptom that brings a man to seek his counsel. "The majority of my clients come to me because they are lonely," he said. "Of course, loneliness is a situation that all people face at some stage in their life. But older men without a partner seem to find loneliness particularly difficult. I see a lot of divorced men, as well as single men who have problems maintaining a long-term relationship."

"How do you help them?" I asked.

"It varies," Jeremy said. "There is no pill in a bottle that cures loneliness. I try to get my clients to actually experience loneliness for what it is, rather than try to manage their distress in self-destructive ways, through drinking, drugs, or destructive social behaviors."

Introverts

Not all men find it troubling to live alone. These men may have an active social life, may date or even be in a committed relationship, but prefer not to share their living space with anyone else. Such men are not necessarily lonely; they simply may be introverts. Introverts are not necessarily antisocial. That is a common misunderstanding. More correctly, extroverts find it stimulating and energizing to be with others; they enjoy going to parties and find it tiresome or boring to be alone. Introverts, by contrast, need time alone to restore their energy. While they may enjoy being with other people, parties and crowds tend to tire them out after a while.

Some men are mixed—part introvert, part extrovert. I am one of those. As a writer and musician, I draw energy from being alone, because that is when I accomplish my creative work. But I also enjoy the company of other people. I like going to parties; I like meeting new friends.

It helps to know which of these three energetic styles—extrovert, introvert, or mixed—best describes you. If you are naturally an introvert but don't know it, you may think there is something wrong with you. The classic bestseller *Quiet: The Power of Introverts in a World That Can't Stop Talking* by Susan Cain is an example of a book that can help introverts better understand themselves.

Ryder the Introvert

Ryder is a software engineer in his forties. Although he has had various relationships with women in his life—some short-term, some longer lasting—he has never lived with a partner, and he has never married.

"I like my independence," Ryder told me. "I've had girlfriends who wanted to move in with me, but I like coming home at the end of a work day to a quiet place where I can just be by myself, watch the news or play video games. My work is intense, and when we are working to a deadline, it can be pretty stressful, so I need that time away from everybody to relax and slow my mind down. I call it 'cave time.' I go into my cave, where everything is just where I put it. If I don't want to tidy up, I don't, and I can just vegetate if I want to. Maybe it's part of working in software. When you're working, your brain is on speed, and you need time to slow it down."

"Have you ever thought of marrying and settling down?"

"Yes," Ryder said, "Sure. I'd like to have kids and all that, but I'd have to find the right woman, which hasn't happened yet, and my whole life would change. I make good money in the work I do, but you're kind of a slave to it. I don't know if I could continue that and take on all the responsibilities of family life."

"So you don't mind being alone?" I asked.

"Hey, I'm an introvert! I was in my thirties before I figured that out. I read some books on introverts and finally realized that's what I was. Until then I thought there was something wrong with me. I went to an introvert support group for a while to learn more. Mostly I learned that I'm perfectly normal. I'm just not the party-hard kind of guy. I've never even been to a rock concert. I couldn't stand the noise and the crowds. I'd rather listen to the same music at home."

"How old are you now?" I said.

"I turn forty-four next month. In the software world, that's old. I've got to compete with twenty-somethings who are whip smart and ambitious as hell. There's ageism in my profession, no question."

"How do you see your life unfolding, say, in the next ten years, when you'll be fifty-four?"

"I try not to think about it," Ryder said. "I don't like the idea of growing old. I like my life the way it is now, but in ten years I don't know if things will still be the same. I'm thinking maybe I should look for a different career, one that gives me more leisure time, where it's okay for me to spend time by myself. But that doesn't go with having a family, so I'm not sure." Ryder sighed. "I guess I'm not ready to think about ten years from now. Not yet."

Sam the Extrovert

Sam had had a successful career as an insurance agent, and as he neared sixty, he had cut his work back to half time so he could travel and also engage in philanthropic activities. His passion was helping disadvantaged youth and refugee children get a good education. Sam was the proverbial "people person"—the glad-hander, the back-slapper, the life of the party, the effusive host. He hardly ever ate at home. He and his wife almost always ate lunch and dinner out, usually in the company of friends or associates.

When I told Sam about this book, he was effusive and encouraging. "A great idea!" he said. "Men need a book like that."

"How about you?" I asked. "Do you think you could use a book about aging for men?"

"Maybe when I get old," Sam laughed. "I'm years away from that."

Sam was rarely alone. Day and night, he was with people. When he traveled, his wife always came with him. He always liked to have stimulation around him. If he was waiting for an appointment, he surfed the net on his phone. At home his entertainment system pumped out an unending stream of music. Sam was a jazz buff and had a big CD library of jazz artists.

I said to Sam, "One thing I have discovered in interviewing men for my book is that they don't like to talk about aging too much. It's something private."

"I wouldn't know," Sam replied. "Never think about it, never talk about it."

"You must think about it sometimes," I said. "You're going to be sixty next year."

"You know what they say," Sam shot back. "Sixty is the new forty."

"Well," I said, "speaking for myself, I find thinking about aging a bit of a lonely business. It's my aging, nobody else's."

We were sitting in Sam's living room, and the sound system had finished its last tune. Sam got up and punched in a new album. "You've got to hear this one," he said. "Young kid in New York, twenty-seven years old. Absolute prodigy on the trumpet.

"I tell you what," Sam continued, as the plaintive sounds of a muted trumpet wafted through his speaker system. "I'm hosting a party next Saturday night—some people in my college scholarship program, mostly guys. Why don't you come by? I'll introduce you around, and you can see if any of the guys are interested in talking about getting old." Sam chuckled. "You might find one or two."

After talking with Sam, I wondered if aging was more accessible to introverts like Ryder, who paid more attention to his inner world. Sam was just not made that way.

We Age Alone

Regardless of whether a man is an introvert, extrovert, or a mixture of the two, in the end, aging is an inward, private thing. Just as my body is unique to me, experienced by no one else, so is my aging particular and private. Aging is an inside game.

In that sense, aging is like being born and dying. At the moment of birth, we emerge from the safety and isolation of our mother's womb. We enter a room full of people—doctors, nurses, a father, and other relatives—and only then do we join the company of other people. Dying is the same. Even though we may be with family and friends at the moment of death, when we disappear into "that good night," we do so without accompaniment. Others bear witness, but we vanish alone.

We can comfort ourselves with the thought that we are years away from that lonely moment, but deep within ourselves the cold fact of death hovers. Aging includes that cold fact. Aging is the downhill slope, and though we don't like to think about what is at the bottom of that decline, in the weeks, months, and years of our aging life, we still feel the pull of its gravity.

Divorce

Men can divorce at any age, but it is a common scenario for men to divorce in midlife, when the children are out of the home, and marital problems that were set aside or ignored while the children were growing up resurface. Such midlife divorces coincide with the onset of aging. For a newly divorced man in midlife, the challenge of creating a new, single life or beginning a relationship with someone new becomes yet one more challenge of aging.

In some ways, divorce favors the husband over the wife; in other ways, not so much. Conventional wisdom holds that, financially speaking, husbands come out better from a divorce than wives. This calculus is changing as women assume a new role as high earners, but by and large, conventional wisdom holds true. Older men can also remain attractive and desirable to potential new partners, since their attractiveness is more tied to money, status, and power. However, divorce can also be more damaging to men than women.[2] Men are more likely to suffer serious depression after a divorce, and they are more disposed to substance abuse.

Gilbert, a recently divorced custom furniture maker in his fifties confirmed these highs and lows. "When we started doing the divorce, my wife wanted the moon. She wanted sole custody, the house, the car, and a piece of my business. Gradually we realized that if we both lawyered up, we would both lose our shirts. So we went into mediation, and things worked out. She did get the house, but I kept my business.

"I've got to tell you, though, being alone after all those years was tough. I started drinking, first wine and then whiskey. I realized if I kept that up, the business would suffer, not to mention my health, so I got some help and stopped cold turkey. At first, I thought it would be easy to date women again, but the whole dating scene has changed. It's all online now, and after a few weird coffee dates, I kind of gave up. So bottom line is, it's been kind of hard.

"Sometimes I even wonder if the divorce was a mistake." Gilbert paused. "Then I think about it and realize of course it was the right thing, but still, sometimes I miss the way things were. Even a lousy marriage has its benefits." Gilbert's voice trailed off.

Gilbert's experience is a typical example of a straight marriage. A gay divorce hews to a different scenario. Since gay marriages have only recently become legal, gay divorces are even newer.

Albert was a gay man who had recently divorced his husband of four years. Albert had just turned fifty.

"It just didn't work out," Albert said. "We were one of the first married gay couples in our community, and there were no models about how it was supposed to work. How was being married different from just living together, which gay men had been doing forever? There was also a lot of social pressure against marriage as a kind of oppressive, hetero institution that didn't have much relevance to the gay experience. We were so excited to have our marriage ceremony and our certificate from the state that said we were legal and recognized. But that wore off after a while, and we both felt that maybe this hitched-for-life thing wasn't right for us.

"Now that the divorce has happened, I'm back to being a single gay man, looking for someone to share my life with. Except I just turned fifty, and I'm competing with guys twenty years younger who are slender and handsome. I'm glad I tried the marriage thing, I felt like a real pioneer at the time, but after those married years of having someone to come home to every night my apartment feels awfully empty."

Searching for a Companion

Single men spend a lot of time searching for a companion—on dating sites, in singles bars, and other venues. Sean, a twice-divorced construction manager still vigorous at age seventy, said, "I'd give anything to have another woman in my life. I've got money, health, a high-status profession—lots of pluses, you'd think. But gals don't want to commit to an older guy. On a dating site, one woman texted me and said, 'You look interesting, but I don't want to be pushing you around in a wheelchair in ten years.'"

"Well, that was hurtful," I said.

"I've heard of worse. Younger guys are used to it, they give as good as they get, but the whole online dating scene is brutal. I'm from another era. When I was in high school and college we actually *dated*. We went out; we did fun things; we got to know each other. Sex happened if it happened, but it wasn't always front and center. I hear about the hookup scene in college now, and I can't relate. The kids say they don't have *time* for a real relationship. What's that about? I keep my hand in online, but I'm also going about things the old-fashioned way, going on group hikes, taking trips to interesting places, getting my buddies to introduce me around. I'm staying positive. Someone right will turn up, I'm sure of it."

Recent studies support Sean's approach. Even though online dating has become the preferred way to meet people (cited by 69 percent of those surveyed in a recent *MIC* poll), that same survey showed that 60 percent of committed couples *actually* met through mutual friends or in some kind of social setting. Single men worn out from the online dating scene can take heart from this.

Rebound Marriage

Connor came to my aging workshop with a woman many years his junior, whom he introduced as Claire, his new wife. Connor had been divorced less than six months when he met Claire. "I thought I would check out this aging thing," Connor said. "But since we've been married, I'm feeling a lot younger."

Connor and Claire seemed happy together, but I sensed a shadow behind Connor's upbeat tone. I'm sure he *felt* ten years younger, but he wasn't. When he reached his mid-seventies, Claire would still be in her mid-fifties. How would that work out?

I have talked to men who rebounded too quickly from a divorce into a new marriage that didn't have a healthy foundation for a long-term relationship. Those marriages ended in another divorce after a year or two. That said, sometimes these second marriages work out well. Connor had followed his divorce with a marriage to a younger woman, and they are the only two people for whom it really matters.

Deep Mind Reflection

In proposing a deep mind reflection for men who are single, divorced, or otherwise alone, let me repeat the comment that the psychologist Jeremy made about how he helps lonely men: "I get men to actually experience loneliness for what it is." That is one objective of this reflection. The other is to make a distinction between being alone and being lonely. Not every man who lives alone is lonely. Introverts enjoy being alone a good bit of the time. But an introvert who is not in relationship, who does not have nourishing friendships, or who actively avoids contact with other people, is not just alone; it's likely that he is also lonely.

For our first reflection on being alone, let's start with the keyword *alone*. *Alone, alone*—you might notice that while you are doing this reflection, you are probably actually alone. Turning your mind's eye inward in the service of knowing yourself better is not a bad thing, even if it is about being alone. So silently intoning the word *alone* in that spirit puts a positive spin on the word and helps clear your mind. The website *Power of Positivity* has articles on this subject: "The 9 Reasons Being Alone is Good for You" and "Being Alone Clears the Mind."

Alone can be a good keyword even if you are married or in a committed relationship. A healthy relationship leaves room for the independence of each partner. If you have a spouse or partner, you might want to spend time inwardly exploring what feelings the word *alone* brings up for you. If you are happy with the relationship, then the word *alone* might evoke another of the "nine reasons for being alone": it strengthens relationships. On the other hand, the word *alone* could bring up the shadow of that happiness, the sobering possibility of what might happen if you lost your partner or grew apart from him or her. Both tonalities of *alone* are valid.

Shifting now to a different situation: if you are recently divorced or have recently broken up with a partner, the word *alone* may evoke the pain of that separation. In that case, sometimes just saying or even thinking the word brings up sadness. In that case the keyword *single* might be more tolerable. *Single* doesn't have the emotional weight and baggage of *alone*. You are just single; that is your situation.

Alone and *single* are two suggestions for a keyword, but there are other possibilities. If you wait in silence and allow your deep mind to propose a keyword that most accurately reflects your present state of mind, it will be interesting to see what word floats to the surface of awareness.

Once you have established your keyword, search for an image that aligns with the feeling of it. There are many images that can come to mind of something solitary—a windswept tree standing alone in a landscape of rolling grassland, a cellphone tower atop a mountain pass, a single ripe peach in a wicker basket. Your image should align with the emotional tone of your aloneness. Not every situation of being alone is unhappy.

What comes to mind for me when I think of being alone comes from a time in college when I liked to ride my bike to a forest preserve where there was a tree-lined reservoir—the water supply for the town I lived in. The forest was not large, and was surrounded by suburban neighborhoods. But if I chose my route carefully, I could walk for an hour without seeing any person or sign of civilization, just the path snaking through the woods and the quiet shoreline of the reservoir. Once I reached it, I could sit by the side of the lake, all by myself, and enjoy the tree-lined vista of the far shore.

As a lifelong meditator and semi-introvert, this vista was calm and restorative for me. I mention my experience to point out that aloneness—even when it comes on the heels of the dissolution of a relationship—can be restorative. Sometimes it is healthy to be alone for a while. Particularly when facing your own advancing years, you need to be sure you don't subsume your private anxieties in a constant swirl of social events and group activities. No one else can do your aging for you. It is your task to master.

If there is actual sadness and loneliness in your solitude, do not try to avoid it. Stay with it as long as you can bear it; it is not a condition to run away from. Turning to face your fears is the essence of courage, and courage is a quality that can restore a man's energy and improve his outlook. You may still be alone, but with courage to support you, you can stand tall and be ready to face the next thing. Remember the adage "every breath, new chances." My Buddhist teacher didn't say "every week" or "every month." There are always new chances, small though they might be, in every moment and every breath. Even a ray of morning sunlight on the mantle can remind you that time and life continue apace, which is just another way to describe what aging is.

7

ILLNESS AND DEATH

Illness and death: that is where aging inexorably leads. We don't like to talk about it. We don't really even like to think about it. Benjamin Franklin tried to make a joke about it, saying that the only certain things in life are death and taxes. Franklin tried to sugar the cookie, but you can't make it sweet. The age you are now today and the age you will be on the day you die create a frame of reference, a temporal hallway with two doors—one starting now and one around the bend, out of sight. The door of today is where we stand, seeing the hallway stretching ahead into the mist. We can't see where the hallway ends—that vista is blurred. But we know, or think we know, what that second door looks like. It looks like nothing. It is black—no more hallway, no tomorrow, nothing beyond. Beyond that second door there is an ill-conceived form of unknowing.

For people of faith whose belief includes an afterlife, that faith offers some shape of what is beyond that door. For those without such a belief, the unknowing beyond that door is unfathomable. Or, as Katherine Hepburn said on her deathbed, when asked about dying, "It's like a long sleep."

Yes, we don't like to think about it, especially if today we are healthy, full of years, and looking forward to a generous lifespan stretching ahead.

The option of not thinking about dying except as something that will happen far off into the future is a relatively recent luxury. Before the discovery of penicillin and other antibiotics in the 1940s, people regularly died suddenly of ailments that today doctors would consider routinely treatable—infections, wounds, pneumonia—not to mention accidents of various kinds. (In the 1800s the leading cause of accidental death in the United States was injury from a horse). Until the 1960s there were few reliable chemotherapy drugs to treat cancer; back then, the very word *cancer* was taboo. I myself survived a type of cancer in the mid-1980s that was 100 percent fatal before a curative regimen was developed in the 1970s.

It wasn't just our own death that could strike without warning. Death from childbirth was a leading cause of death for young women. Children were "taken off" by diseases such as diphtheria, whooping cough, and measles. Today there are vaccines for these killers; and, strangely, a new anti-vaccine movement is rising up with a kind of amnesia for those earlier dire times. Polio used to strike legions of children every summer; parents lived in mortal fear of it.

So we live in a time bubble in which illness and death can be kept safely at arm's length—though, obviously pandemic life has punctured this safety bubble for many, especially older adults with compromised health. Still, denial about the harsh reality can keep us complacent and happy about our lifespan chances. From one point of view this is a good thing. Who would want to voluntarily dwell on misfortune unless it were necessary? From another perspective, though, it may be useful to remember that as we age, our bodies are slowly losing their miraculous ability to self-repair. Lifestyle illnesses are the slow killers these days—obesity, heart disease, diabetes, and lung cancer—and these possibilities need regular tending and attention to be held at bay.

Another point: the time bubble of our complacency may be smaller than we think. The world is warming, and insect-borne diseases like dengue fever and malaria are moving north out of the tropics. The antibiotic miracle that began with penicillin is also showing signs of waning. Some diseases from an earlier time, such as tuberculosis and even some sexually transmitted diseases, are becoming resistant to every available medicine. We are also seeing a proliferation of auto-immune diseases.

The aging body, in short, demands attention. As one friend of mine who loved to work on classic cars used to say, "When you get older, you need to do more and more chassis maintenance."

When I was young, I used to wonder what it was about older people—such as my grandparents—that made them seem somber and serious, at least to my childish eye. Now that I am one of those older people, I think it was because of the number of funerals they had been to. Noted political commentator Michael Kinsley, in an article for the *New Yorker*, once quoted an actuarial statistic that has stayed with me.[1] The median age, he said, when you find that you go to more than one funeral in a given year is sixty-two. I'm seventy-two, and I've been to enough funerals in the last ten years to know that this statistic seems right.

Even if you and your loved ones are perfectly healthy, if you are older than sixty-two, the funerals have probably begun for you—or will soon. Perhaps you may not yet have noticed the accumulated weight of watching your friends depart this earth one by one, or maybe you have but do not dwell on it. But this is the reality of what aging is. As the weight of these departures increases, their shadow grows, and with each passing year, it becomes an increasing part of who we are.

The shadow of grief that slumbers under the radar can suddenly break through. And then the tears may come. When I woke up from my encephalitic coma, I was emotionally volatile and cried all the time. Even the smallest setback would cause me to burst into tears. This was disturbing to me. I said to my psychiatrist, "I feel like I'm going crazy."

His replied, "No, you're just experiencing emotions. Those emotions will help you heal."

I think my reaction was typical of men my age. It was not just the belief that men don't cry. I just didn't feel right inside. Once in therapy I blurted out, "I feel like a woman!"—a confession that embarrassed me. I hadn't learned yet that vulnerability is not weakness; it is strength.

The problem-solving skills of the intellect are ill-adapted to cope with these situations. The reality is that with each passing year, the chances of one partner of an aging couple becoming seriously ill increases. This is why financial advisors consistently advise purchasing long-term care insurance, and why the premiums for such insurance rise markedly after age seventy.

If serious illness strikes, emotions can overwhelm a man, leaving him feeling helpless and without resources. My hope is that reading this chapter—and practicing the reflection at the end—will raise male readers' awareness of this issue and make them more prepared if a crisis occurs.

The Death of My Sister

During the writing of this book, my sister died. She had already been ill for over ten years, ever since she was diagnosed with ovarian cancer at the age of sixty-four. I had lost two close friends to ovarian cancer already, and neither of them lasted longer than three years. My sister had already beaten those odds. They say that siblings are connected in a deep way—two souls from the same womb. She was my only sibling, five years older. I had known her all my life, from the earliest days of our childhood together. No one knew her better than I did.

I remember when she first called me, her voice trembling, to tell me she had a large tumor in her pelvis. I listened calmly, trying to reassure her—though having survived cancer myself, many decades before, I knew what the diagnosis was likely to be. As soon as I got off the phone, my heart sank. A sense of vertigo and anxiety washed over me. I felt her panic as my panic. I remembered that moment long ago when I sat in my own doctor's office, and he told me I had a cancerous tumor in my abdomen. I was thirty-five at the time. Then it was like being hit by a freight train. And now it was happening to my sister.

The thing about a life-threatening illness like cancer is that it is inescapable. It doesn't matter how strong or courageous you are. It doesn't matter that it isn't necessarily a death sentence. Many people recover from cancer; I did. It is simply that there is an inexorable line that the diagnosis forces you to cross. Before that moment you were normal and ordinary, trekking through your daily routines, planning for the next day, the next week or month. But once you cross that line, all of that is swept away as though by a hurricane. At whatever age you are when that hurricane hits, you suddenly feel quite old. You find you have very little future that you can count on. You are in a land of shadow, a terrain of darkness, and feel as though you have been struck blind.

If you are not the patient, you also feel particularly helpless. When you are the patient, as my sister was, at least you have things to do, medical tests to go to, surgery to schedule, specialists to see. These appointments and activities give you purpose and provide a sense of forward movement and hope. When you are the friend or a relative, as I was, the helplessness is constant. There is really nothing you can do except think about it all the time, occasionally forget that you have been thinking about it, and then have it suddenly hit you again.

When faced with this sort of dire news, the mind grasps for any lifeline. My first thought was, *I had cancer, and I was cured, so she too can be cured*. (That turned out not to be true). My second thought was, *Okay, this is a problem that can be solved. Let's get to work on it.* (No, it could not be solved. I repeat: it was an illness that had no cure.) My third thought—not a thought, really, but a feeling—was despair. *My sister is going to die, and there's nothing I can do about it.*

As it happened, my sister kept beating the odds. After twelve years she was still going strong. She endured many bouts of debilitating chemotherapy. She tried various alternative treatments. She had surgeries. She took on her cancer as an all-encompassing project and faced it with uncommon courage and creativity. She continued teaching music, she led an active life, she traveled, and she continued to prevail as her place on the bell curve of cancer survival kept getting pushed farther out.

I walked with her on this epic journey as her loving brother, encouraging her, letting her know of new medicines and treatments I had heard about. I became her partner in illness as her body aged from the cancer and the toxic treatments for it. Perhaps you have a friend, a relative, or a spouse or partner who is going through something similar. This kind of illness is a different kind of aging, a kind that happens in the "valley of the shadow of death." You can't take a vacation from that shadow. You can't get a facelift, a belly tuck, a new vitamin, or weight-loss regimen to make it go away. You just have to keep putting one foot in front of the other, which is the way life always is anyway, though usually we manage to think otherwise.

The time came when my sister was actually dying. Her children and grandchildren had come for one last visit, and following that, she decided to stop eating and drinking—which had become uncomfortable for her anyway. Though she was slowly wasting away and growing more tired, she was still pretty pain free. Her comment during this time was, "Well, I've been through natural childbirth, now I get to experience natural death."

I hoped that when her death came, that it would be peaceful. However, a good friend of mine who was one of the founders of the hospice movement told me once, "Lew, the one thing to remember about dying is that it never happens the way you think or hope it's going to. It's different for every person, and you can't choose how it will be."

In her last few days, things changed, and my sister experienced great pain. She took a lot of morphine to cope with it. She died in her sleep.

We can't choose how we will die or how we will age. We are always aging beings, and there are as many different ways to age as there are people. I can't choose which way it will be for me— whether I will remain healthy, become ill, or fall and break my leg. I can only choose how to deal with it as it comes.

Jan

Jan was a healthy man in his early fifties, athletic and fit. He played a low-handicap game of golf and enjoyed tennis and pickup basketball. He had never had a serious illness or injury and said that his doctor had told him he had the heart and lungs of a man half his age.

He was vacationing at a lakeside resort in the mountains with his girlfriend, paddling a canoe on the lake, when he began to feel short of breath. He passed it off as a reaction to the high altitude, and thought no more of it. However, when they returned to their room and went to dinner, the shortness of breath persisted. His girlfriend wondered if it could be allergies; her allergies sometimes made her feel short of breath. But Jan didn't know of any allergies that he had.

By the next morning he was definitely feeling unwell. It was hard for him even to walk up the stairs to their room. His girlfriend suggested that he check in at the local medical clinic, but Jan resisted. "There's nothing wrong with me," he said. "Just the thin mountain air."

But by midafternoon he felt a heaviness in his chest, and his legs were wobbly. He decided to go to the clinic after all. At the clinic, the nurse took his vital signs and blanched. "Your blood pressure hardly registers," she said. "You're lucky you haven't passed out. You need to see the doctor right away."

The doctor came in, took his blood pressure again and listened to his heart. "Your heartbeat is weak and irregular," the doctor said. "You need to go to the hospital right away and get this checked out. We don't have the equipment here to do a full heart workup. I think we should call an ambulance."

"An ambulance?" said Jan incredulously. "You've got to be kidding. My girlfriend can drive me."

When they got in the car, Jan decided, instead of going to the local hospital, to drive back home—a three-hour drive—so he could be seen by doctors he knew. He kept his voice reassuringly light, but for the first time, he was inwardly concerned. What could be wrong? He had just had a physical, and his heart was fine.

At the big-city hospital, they wheeled Jan into a room full of equipment and did a high-tech scan of his chest. He lay there on the gurney while the technicians analyzed the result. Suddenly the door opened, and the room was full of people.

A grey-haired doctor leaned over him. "I'm Dr. Singh, the head of cardiology here. You have a major blood clot in your heart and at least ten small ones in your lungs. I'm amazed you didn't collapse on the way here. If that clot breaks free and goes to your brain, you could have a stroke or even die. As it is, your heart is quite compromised. It's only working at 20 or 30 percent."

Jan, now truly alarmed, lifted himself up to reply but the doctor firmly pushed him back onto the gurney. "Don't move. We have to get you hooked up to some special equipment and watch that clot around the clock."

"What can you do for it?" Jan asked. "Aren't there medicines that can fix it?"

"There are," Dr. Singh said, "but that clot is so large that breaking it up could make it even more dangerous, creating many smaller clots. Once we get you stabilized, I'll come back, and we can discuss treatment options."

Jan, a naturally gregarious person, chatted up all the nurses and other specialists that flitted in and out of his room. Lying flat on his back, he didn't feel so bad, but he was surrounded by complex equipment that emitted intimidating beeps, clicks, and buzzes.

In the early evening Dr. Singh returned. "We've gotten you stabilized but that clot could break up or move at any time. We have two options. We could take you upstairs to surgery tonight and do open-heart surgery to try to remove the clot. Or we could use clot-busting medicine to try to dissolve it."

"Which is the least dangerous?" Jan said.

"They're both dangerous," Dr. Singh replied. "The clot could move while you are on the operating table and kill you. And if we use the clot-busting medication there is a 30 percent chance you could have a major stroke."

Jan's brain raced. He had never before been in a situation where he had to quickly make up his mind with his very life on the line. "Will I be awake while the clot-busting drug is working?"

"You have to be," Dr. Singh said. "We're going to need to check to every fifteen minutes to make sure you haven't had a stroke."

"Then I'll go with the medicine," Jan said. "If I'm going to die, I'd rather be awake when it happens."

As night came on and Jan lay in bed being tended by several nurses who indeed checked his vital signs and alertness every fifteen minutes, Jan had time to reflect on the sudden turn his life had taken. A few days before, he was vital and healthy, full of energy and enjoying life. Now he was possibly on the brink of death or severe incapacitation. Nevertheless, he was not depressed. Perhaps it was just wishful thinking, but he had a firm conviction that he would get through this, the medicine would work, and that in no time he would be back to his old life.

"Ready for your stroke tests?" Tony had come in, the neurological technician who was assigned to check on Jan for signs of stroke.

Jan knew the drill by heart. He closed his eyes, touched his finger to his nose, counted from one to ten, read the eye chart from across the room backward and forward—the tests went on.

"Okay," Tony said brightly when they were finished. "No stroke. See you in fifteen."

Jan's optimism was rewarded. He did not die. He did not have a stroke. In a few days he was discharged from the hospital—"good as new," Dr. Singh said—no sign that he had been through hell and back except his arms, which were black and blue from all the blood they had to draw.

At first, Jan told me, he was floating on a cloud, elated that he had gotten his life back with no apparent damage. That mood lasted for a couple of weeks. Then, as he was getting on a plane to fly East to visit his family, he suddenly felt a sense of panic, which persisted throughout the flight. On the surface, his intellect had concluded that he had dodged a huge bullet, his good luck held, and all was well. But his deep mind knew that back in the hospital he could have died, and he saw a plane trip as a new dire threat. Jan felt as though he had fallen off a cliff.

"For a couple of months after that panic attack on the plane I felt pretty shaken up," Jan said. "I'm me, still the upbeat, optimistic guy who is pretty sure he can beat anything. But some part of me now knows different. That trip to the hospital was a wake-up call, and I know now that any time, any day, it could happen again.

"I guess I would say I'm more serious now, more grateful and also more careful. I'm not an old man, not by a long shot, but now I'm not a young man either. The tick-tock of life is catching up with me. Some part of me gets that this is just how it is, and some part of me is pissed as hell."

Deep Mind Reflection: Illness and Wellness

Any reflection about illness and death is bound to be challenging. Your deep mind may not quite know what to do with the feelings these words evoke. *Death* is a pretty loaded word. You might find focusing on it difficult and depressing. On the other hand, there are religious contexts in which meditation on death is encouraged. Medieval Christian monks practiced *memento mori,* the remembrance of death, as a focus of religious practice. A biblical passage expresses it this way: "In all thy works be mindful of thy last end." The Buddha also taught the reality of old age, sickness, and death as a deep truth of human life well worth pondering. For religious professionals committed to deep spiritual work, these approaches may be appropriate. But in the context of our exploration of aging, I think we need a lighter touch.

The words *illness* and *wellness* are more manageable, I think, than *death.* After all, we are all familiar with illness and injury. Certainly, by the time you are fifty, you have dealt with multiple instances of both. Even if you were blessed—as Jan was before his blood clot—with an illness-free adulthood, sooner or later major illness is inescapable. We all have to deal with it.

So, let's begin with *illness* as our keyword. *Illness, illness.* Allow yourself to remember times you have been ill, or when someone close to you has been ill. At the same time, form a picture in your mind of where you were—lying in bed at home or in the hospital—and how you felt. Miserable, probably. We tend to forget what a gift wellness is until we are ill, and then we wish nothing better than to be well again.

That is why, for this reflection, I would like you to incorporate a second keyword: *wellness. Illness, wellness, illness, wellness.* Let your mind consider both words. They are the two sides of the one coin of life. Mostly we are well, sometimes we are ill. As we age, we will be well somewhat less often and ill somewhat more often. Illness in this context includes injury. Even a healthy man is subject to bodily wear and tear as he ages—be it tennis elbow, a sprained ankle, a pulled or torn muscle, or a bad back. Injuries—especially sports injuries—are one topic that aging men do readily talk about among themselves: what happened, how it happened, how it feels, what the doctor says, when it will heal. The older you get, the more illness and wellness will be on your radar. We're on the lookout for anything that impacts our wellness—a state that starts to feel more fragile with each passing year.

As you contemplate the two keywords, *illness* and *wellness,* form an image of an illness or injury you had that you completely recovered from, and recall what it felt like to be well again. It could be a broken leg from a skiing accident, for example. You were in pain, the doctors put you in an uncomfortable cast, you hobbled around on crutches for a couple of months, you were miserable, and so on. After the cast came off, you had to go to rehab. Your leg was weak, and you had to do tiresome physical exercises every day to get your strength back.

But finally, it was over. The leg was strong again—good as new, you thought. You "got back on the horse," went back up to the slopes, and had a satisfying weekend of skiing on your good-as-new leg.

Whatever injury or affliction you pick out of your own experience, this type of reflection has a deeper purpose. It reminds you that your body, aging though it might be, still has miraculous healing powers. Any doctor will tell you that medicine and physical therapy only go so far; the body itself does most of the healing. How do the bones know how to knit and regrow? How do the weakened muscles know in what fashion to build back new fiber and tissue? Your body is gifted with healing wisdom; if you stop to think about it, it's like magic.

The recommendations you can read about concerning ways to stay healthy rely on this body magic. For example, walking thirty minutes a day, 150 minutes a week, reduces the risk of heart attack and stroke by 30 percent—that's what current medical knowledge says. This kind of moderate exercise has also proven to be the best preventative against mental decline and dementia. There is no miracle drug for dementia, at least not yet—drug companies have been trying for years to come up with the right elixir. In the meantime, simple exercise, done regularly, acts as a bulwark against that one major fear as we age—dementia.

This is probably because the body has evolved to move, and even in old age, any moving you do keeps you strong. Until the age of modern transportation, human beings walked everywhere. You have the same body that men had five thousand or fifty thousand years ago. "Illness and wellness" as a reflection connects us to these ancient ancestors, who were physically active up until the moment they perished.

Next, see if you can also turn this reflection on illness and wellness into a contemplation of gratitude. We tend to take wellness for granted, as the normal, default state of affairs, but, particularly as we grow older, a day of feeling healthy and whole is also grounds for a day of gratitude. Gratitude is also the best antidote for any feelings of sadness and loss that come up as you meditate on your fragility and mortality. This is especially important if you or a loved one are dealing with a chronic or degenerative disease like Parkinson's, multiple sclerosis, emphysema, or early dementia. Faced with these challenges, it's especially hard to generate feelings of gratitude. But remember what one of my Buddhist teachers used to say: "The ultimate fact is that you are here, right now." Being here is the ultimate gift, and no matter what the challenge, you can say—like my friend the psychiatrist—"There is always something you can do."

There is indeed something, even if it is just to take another breath, take another sip of water, take another footstep, or steal another glance out the window to appreciate the sunny day.

Illness and wellness are the fraternal twins of aging. Where there is wellness, there is the shadow of illness. Where there is illness, there is the possibility of wellness—or, in the case of chronic conditions or irreversible decline, the chance of an occasional respite, however modest.

8

HEALTH—PHYSICAL, EMOTIONAL, AND SPIRITUAL

Books and articles on aging tend to focus on physical health. They offer lots of practical advice about vitamins, exercise, smoking, drinking, blood pressure, virility, heart attacks, diabetes, and stroke. I'm not sure how much all this well-meaning advice gets through to the typical man. By the time a man is in his fifties, his lifestyle habits are ingrained and are difficult to change. Most men I know try to abide by some of these principles of healthy lifestyle, but I'm not sure how many actually succeed at all of it.

My own health focus is diet; I have a prediabetic condition, and I need to avoid sugars and white carbs and keep my weight below a certain number. But I also love to eat. I love potatoes and white bread, butter and brie. I always seem to be about six to eight pounds heavier than my ideal target weight. I do walk thirty minutes six or seven days a week; I'm sure that helps. But the bottom line is that it's hard to stay healthy as you age. It takes work and the kind of self-discipline that requires sustained energy.

I could compile a whole chapter about lifestyle advice. I have done a lot of research for my own benefit and know all the principles. But I would be repeating material that can be found in many places. In any case, these kinds of physical health concerns—the focus of a large, profitable industry—are only one dimension of the aging process. There are other aspects of well-being that are equally important—emotional health and spiritual health. When it comes to physical health—diet, exercise, physical exams, taking medications—men can be placed on a bell curve of compliance. At one end are men who disregard or ignore all these health practices entirely, floating along in a cocoon of denial until some health crisis wakes them up. At the other are men who follow them to the letter. While not giving short shrift to taking care of the physical body, this chapter focuses on the emotional and spiritual aspects of health.

Worry

A recent article in *Time* magazine reports that on the whole, older people are better at dealing with major stress than younger ones—probably because we have had a lot more practice at it.[1] At the same time, the stresses that come with aging are more chronic. They don't resolve easily and tend to dog us month after month. Financial stress would be one example; health worries another. Some men worry a lot; others little or not at all.

Jordan was on the ignore-it-all end of the bell curve.

"You have high blood pressure," the doctor said to Jordan. "Dangerously high."

"No, I'm good, doc," Jordan replied. "I just had three cups of coffee before I came over here. That's why I'm buzzed. I'm fine."

"No, you're not," the doctor said. "You could keel over any moment. You need to go to the hospital right now."

"I'll be okay," Jordan insisted. "No worries."

This true story shows the power of denial even when faced with a life-threatening condition. This kind of denial may seem illogical, but Jordan was not just being stubborn. He was in denial, which meant that he simply could not hear what his doctor was telling him. That is how denial works; it blocks the mind from processing something it doesn't want to hear or is afraid to hear.

Jordan was one of those people who has learned to deal with life problems through denial. On first meeting him, I was struck with his easygoing and happy-go-lucky attitude. For those of us who worry a lot, Jordan's what-me-worry constitution might seem like a blessing. However, this story about his high blood pressure illustrates the dark side of denial. Jordan's blithe dismissal of his doctor's warning could have led to a serious health crisis, even death. The doctor eventually convinced Jordan to go to the hospital, but even this scare would probably not change Jordan's denial-friendly approach to life. It was too deeply ingrained.

There is a stereotype about aging, pushed by media and advertising, that it is supposed to be relaxed and carefree—hence the term *golden years.* I don't know who it was who coined this term; maybe an advertising executive. Personally, I find the phrase rather cloying. The aging years can't be characterized by any particular color. Aging is complex and multi-hued. Certainly, there are some life problems that you don't have to worry about as you get older—getting your high school son or daughter into a good college, for example. But other worries replace them.

Then there are worries that never go away. For example, no matter how old your children are, you never stop worrying about them. My son is forty-five. We often don't hear from him for weeks at a time, but we think about him often and are always pleased when we hear from him. Your children are gone from your home, but never from your heart.

Another chronic worry as we age is money. Unless you are independently wealthy, you need to worry about money. That need never goes away. In fact, the minute you stop drawing a paycheck and are reliant on Social Security and whatever nest egg you have set aside, your money worries continue—perhaps even increase. On a fixed income, there are no new savings accounts to raid or higher-paying jobs to take if a crisis comes. It's nice to imagine that we could live to be ninety or older in good health, but not if that means we are going to run out of money.

Worry affects your health in a number of ways. For one thing, it disturbs your sleep, and getting enough sleep is essential for older adults. Worry drives up your blood pressure and puts a strain on your heart. It can also lead to destructive behaviors like drinking too much or taking drugs.

I am the opposite of happy-go-lucky Jordan. I have always been a worrier, always looking ahead for possible difficulties or surprises, and developing contingency plans to deal with them. This personal style has served me well in software. A good software developer always anticipates what might go wrong and puts contingent logic in place in case it does. In software, Murphy's Law rules—the principle that anything that *can* go wrong *will* go wrong. Many times I have had to pull an all-nighter, working to solve a critical client problem in time for them to open for business the next morning.

My worrying nature was not an advantage, however, once we decided to sell the house and move. There were just too many decisions—large and small—to be made, and too many unknowns for my programmer's brain to keep up with. Whether it was a small decision to keep or discard a cherished old book, or whether it was deciding to spend a bundle to remodel the bathroom, my brain was in constant overload. This state of affairs followed me to bed. I would wake up in the middle of the night and find these problems running like frightened mice through my brain, seemingly intractable in the dead of night.

My wife, Amy, doesn't have my kind of brain. She doesn't worry about things much before they happen. What's more, while I tend to talk through each problem—often repeating myself as I go—Amy keeps her concerns to herself. Many times, I didn't know what she was thinking, or whether she was worrying about the same things I was (often she was, but in her own quiet way).

Talkative worrier and quiet worrier—the two of us actually made a good team. We supported each other's respective problem-solving styles. But we still worried, and it wasn't fun to plod through each day with a furrowed brow, subsisting on five hours sleep.

Stress

Worry and stress go together. Worry causes stress, and stressful situations cause us to worry. Worry, because it is largely self-generated, can be managed to some extent. Stress from outside just lands in your lap like an unwelcome cat.

When I told my personal physician that we were selling our house and moving to a new town, he told me that next to the death of a spouse or close relative, moving to a new home caused the highest stress of any life event. When I added that my sister was dying, he replied, "That's a real double whammy."

When you are younger, moving is not a big deal; you move all the time. You move away from home to college, you move from college to your first apartment, you move to a bigger apartment or a first home, and so on. Typically, you are so busy living your young life that you hardly notice the stress.

Amy and I thought back to the last time we moved—thirty years ago we moved from a small rental home to a larger home we had purchased—and realized that back then we were so busy at our respective jobs that we couldn't remember much of it. We did it more or less on autopilot. We did remember that we had only a fraction of the furniture and possessions that we had now.

This time, with more time on our hands, we were acutely conscious of every aspect of the move. We knew we had to do it, we wanted to do it, and we planned what we thought were all the steps. What we were not prepared for was the sense of uprootedness; the loss of long-established routines; the difficult discussions to keep a thing or let go of it; the physical difficulty of packing, lifting, loading, and unloading; and the toll it took on our aging bodies. Most of all we didn't anticipate the combined effect of all these things on our sense of composure—the drumbeat of hourly, daily stress and the difficulty of getting a good night's sleep.

Our first move was to temporary quarters so the painters and contractors could tear things up in our old house without our being there. By the time we packed boxes and suitcases for the temporary move, our furniture and possessions were gone into storage, the house was empty, and the home where we had lived comfortably for thirty years was already becoming a memory. Since renting an apartment was impractical for such a short time period, we chose a nearby extended-stay hotel with a full kitchen, living room, and bedroom. It seemed ideal for our purposes. We got the reduced winter rate, and we could move in with minimal possessions, keep an eye of how the remodel was going, and continue our life as temporary vagabonds.

It seemed ideal—in theory—except for the fact that it was noisy and not very private. After a few days there, I began to feel irritable. Our room overlooked a swimming pool, and all day it was full of children splashing and making noise. Just as each day wound down, and the children were, at long last, being called in by their parents for dinner, the late check-ins started to arrive. Since we were on the second floor of three, instead of welcome quiet, these new arrivals produced a whole new source of noise. The hotel was old, and the walls and floors were not well insulated, so the thumping of dropped suitcases and booted feet kept us up, sometimes late into the night. Once a troupe of college girls checked in above us, and from the sound of it appeared to be continuously running back and forth from the living room to the bedroom—right above our bedroom—until three in the morning.

I'm unusually sensitive to noise, but I did my best to cope. I found special earplugs highly rated for sound reduction. Those helped some, though while I was wearing them, I couldn't hear anything Amy said to me. When the earplugs weren't strong enough for me to sleep, I found a white noise app for my phone that played a variety of soothing sounds such as croaking frogs or a running creek. I learned from Google that these apps were just the thing for travel warriors in airplanes and hotel rooms. I had, it seemed, joined their number.

On good days, this state of affairs was tolerable. On bad days, trapped by the cacophony, I wanted to shriek like the kids in the pool. Night after night I couldn't sleep. After a couple of weeks, I was a nervous wreck, at the very time when I needed all my marbles to deal with the house remodel.

I felt rather ashamed of myself. The kids in the pool were having a great time, and when I found myself wishing them gone, I felt like a crotchety old Scrooge. This was not the kind and compassionate person that I imagined myself to be. We'd chosen to be here and needed this kind of lodging. In fact, we discovered that there were families in the hotel who had been victims of the huge fires in the previous year that had destroyed two thousand homes a few miles to the north. For them, having a motel room was a huge gift. They would gladly have put up with anything for a place to live. Noise was the least of their concerns.

And here I was feeling sorry for myself because, by my own choice, I was no longer living in a quiet home on a quiet street. I understood intellectually that I should be grateful. But I couldn't help it—I was still stressed out.

I saw these inadequacies as a blow to my self-esteem. Wasn't I a strong person? Hadn't I overcome worse crises? After all, in my software business I had dealt with all manner of crises, including times when I didn't think I could make payroll and was a couple of billing cycles away from going out of business. Why was I having such a hard time dealing with something so mundane as moving?

A psychiatrist friend told me not to be so hard on myself. It happens to the best of us. "All it takes is a bad case of the flu or a big financial reversal, and all our altruism goes out the window," he said. "It doesn't take much for any of us to regress to a point where selfish needs come to the fore. It's the survival brain at work."

Undoubtedly you have had periods in your own life when some stress like this has caused you to falter. Take heart; it does not mean you are any less of a person, any less capable or strong, then you were before. It just means you are human. Faced with stress, your brain does what it needs to do to help you survive. Do what you need to do. Don't be proud. If you need sleeping pills, take them. If you need earplugs, wear them. If you need an occasional tranquilizer, don't worry—just don't take to many of them. Just don't self-medicate with too much alcohol or other harmful drugs. Going down that slippery slope is far worse than the stress that started you slipping.

Later, after our house had sold and we were out from under, we had dinner with Keith and Jennifer, a couple our age, who had also remodeled their house, sold it, and bought a new one to retire in. We exchanged our tales of woe.

Jennifer listened to our story, nodded and said, "That's exactly how it was for me. I couldn't sleep. I needed sleeping pills. I couldn't turn my brain off, there were so many things, large and small, to be thinking about. I felt terrible. I wasn't at all like myself. For the first time in my life, I felt as though I simply couldn't cope."

It was helpful for me to hear that confirmation. I would guess the experience we had had is actually pretty common. It is sobering to realize that the adult masteries you think you have well in hand can slip from your grasp under stress. I already mentioned that, on the whole, older adults handle stress well—but perhaps not the kind of stress we were under, which was so physical. The lesson we learned is that as aging people, our stamina and our resilience can buckle when things get tough.

Now I feel like myself again, and the next time we have to face a challenge like that—if there is a next time—I'll try to remember not to beat myself up too much. It was tough, but I think on balance we did okay.

Drinking and Substance Abuse

For some men, high stress can lead to bad lifestyle choices, which can markedly affect their health—even kill them. We are currently in the midst of a massive crisis of opioid substance abuse. In 2018 opioid overdoses caused 68,000 deaths, and many times that number of near-deaths, calls to the emergency room, family tragedy, and ruined lives. Some of this abuse begins with treatment for chronic physical pain such as a bad back—a common ailment among older men. Compounding the problem is the ready availability of these addictive drugs and the ease with which doctors can prescribe them or the internet can supply them.

We now know that drug companies have flooded society with billions of readily available and highly profitable pills. A bottle of oxycodone is now as easy to get as a pint of whiskey and nearly as cheap. This state of affairs means that what was once garden-variety stress can now lead some men to the nightmare of addiction. Add to this the easiest-to-obtain stress-reducing drug of all— alcohol—and you have a situation in which it takes a strong will to face serious stress without chemical help. A recent *New York Times* article reported than one in ten older adults binge drinks.[2] We think of binge-drinking as something just college students do, but clearly that is not true.

Scott, age fifty-eight, was a recently retired and divorced software engineer who was now working on his own, developing an iPhone app. Scott was overweight, a smoker both of cigarettes and marijuana, who ate most of his meals out. He also liked two or three glasses of wine for dinner plus a whiskey—"so I can sleep," he told me.

I asked Scott if he was aware that his lifestyle choices put him at risk for a variety of illnesses.

"Yeah, sure," Scott said. "I know that. I'm working on it. I've cut back."

I had heard those responses before. When it came to his health, Scott was in denial, and no amount of well-meaning advice from me was likely to reach him. His brain circuits were blocking my words.

Scott was on the edge of addiction and, with any additional strain, could topple in. As a college student, he told me, he had been a regular pot smoker. During his software career—which demanded a sharp mind—he limited his pot smoking to weekends, but now he had taken it up on a daily basis.

"How often do you toke up?" I asked. "Every day?"

Scott shook his head. "Not *every* day," he said. "Hey, it's not addictive. Weed is harmless, right? And now it's legal."

Yes, marijuana is not *physically* addictive, but together with his drinking, Scott's drug and alcohol consumption showed a troubling pattern.

If your lifestyle and substance abuse patterns resemble Scott's to any extent, take action now, before it's too late. Drinking too much as you age is not good, either for health or happiness. An eighty-year longitudinal study at Harvard about long-term causes of happiness discovered, among other things, that "those who lived longer and enjoyed sound health avoided smoking and alcohol in excess."[3] Men tend to think that they are strong enough to "handle" drugs and alcohol and that they will know when too much is too much. I knew a middle-aged artist who told me, "I know exactly how much alcohol I can drink before it's time to stop. I'm in control."

Correction: he's not. He was already an alcoholic, one in denial. Being strong has nothing to do with it. Addictive substances change every cell in your body—permanently—and push them to crave more. Be smarter than your cells and go cold turkey while you can. Get help if you need it.

Spiritual Health

You don't often see references to spiritual health in relation to aging. It's not even clear what spiritual health might mean in an aging context. That's one reason why I wrote the book *Aging as a Spiritual Practice*. In that book I tried to provide a definition and context for the spiritual aspects of aging.

In developing my vocabulary for that book, I used the word *spiritual* rather than *religious* because I didn't want to limit my discussion to any particular religious faith or belief system. For me, *spiritual* means that aspect of our life that deals with fundamental questions about existence. What is our purpose on this earth? What core values should we live by? As we grow older and have experienced all the things that happened to happen, where are we headed? And what will happen when we die? What about the loved ones we leave behind?

I know many men who would not feel comfortable talking about any of these questions. To some men, talking about them seems to violate the masculine principle to stand strong and maintain a taciturn demeanor. In other words, rest in what you know and don't admit what you don't know. These fundamental questions, to many men, imply uncertainty, weakness, or doubt. That said, I believe that most men do enter this terrain of fundamental questions in the privacy of their own thoughts. These questions are all central to aging—especially when we ask, "Reflecting on the life I have lived, what did it all mean? How do I feel about it as I march into the twilight of my own time?"

This reflection belongs here in a chapter on health because our bodies and minds are not just machines, to be kept well oiled and smoothly humming for as long as possible. We are also all souls on a journey, and without a clear picture of where the journey leads and where it ends, the rest of the system is wanting in meaning. In medical terms, we can become anxious or depressed, but those psychological diagnoses do not, in my view, really capture the feeling of being lost, confused, or at sea. There is a psychological component, for sure, but the main issue is existential and spiritual—realms that no medical diagnosis can capture.

This is the spiritual conundrum of growing old, and it needs tending as much as our blood pressure or cholesterol. Whether or not spiritual questions have come forward thus far in your life, aging will bring them forward—if not now, then presently. It's good to be prepared for them and even to welcome them, because the question of life's meaning and death's presentiment—even if your actual death is many years off—is key to making growing old a genuine "golden age" in the sense that gold represents the most precious thing.

Deep Mind Reflections

I focus this chapter's reflections on two topics: stress and the spiritual. Both are foundational, and both are within our grasp and our personal control. By managing stress, we forestall or minimize many health problems, and when we bring into view the big questions, we can be better prepared to face with equanimity the steady march of days, months, and years.

These days many articles about managing stress include the advice to try meditation. This is not bad advice as far as it goes, but the meditation guidance typically offered is usually some kind of calming technique. I taught Buddhist meditation for many years, and during that time, I learned that effective meditation cannot really be taught as a mere technique. Meditation is an art in the way that hitting a baseball is an art. You can't really learn it from a book; you need someone who knows how it is done to initiate you into the feeling of it. These reflections I teach at the end of each chapter are something like that. They initiate you into the art of focusing the mind not on some outside object but on the mind itself.

With that in mind, let's start by taking up the issue of stress. Begin by bringing up the keyword *stress* and letting it linger in awareness. *Stress, stress.* Stress has weight, like a barbell or a heavy book. It sinks rather than rises. *Stress, stress.* At this point, some specific thoughts or images may come to mind about stresses you are dealing with right now or have dealt with recently. Let these come and go, but see if you can stay focused on the keyword until a picture comes to mind.

Where is this picture located and how are you interacting with it? If it is a heavy stone, are you straining to hold it? Is it balanced on your shoulder? Is it leaning against your foot? Stress is not pleasant, so your key image should reflect that feeling tone.

Your key image could also be a health issue you are dealing with. Maybe you're having some pain in your chest or queasiness in your stomach. Do you ignore it? Do you surf the web for your symptoms? Do you take aspirin? When do you call the doctor? If you're like many men, you put off calling the doctor. Suppose you go, and it turns out to be nothing? Embarrassing! Embarrassment may be part of your reluctance, but one of the reasons men die of heart attacks (as I've been told by emergency room doctors) is that they don't go to the ER soon enough when they have chest pain. The ER doctors all say, "When in doubt, go!" Don't die because you want to be a tough guy.

When I do this reflection myself and search for a picture, what comes to mind is our local emergency room. My wife recently tripped and fell and cut her brow. She bled a lot, and I had to take her to the ER. To me, the cut looked minor, and I hoped it just needed a few stitches. But once upon a time, when encephalitis overtook me, I was taken to an ER, and it turned out I was close to dying. I remembered that. Suppose she wasn't going to be okay? Suppose she had hit her head harder than we thought and had a concussion? Suppose she had internal bleeding in her brain? Over the years, I had picked up just enough medical knowledge to scare myself.

So that was my key image: sitting in the ER examining room next to Amy while she held a bloody towel to her forehead, waiting for the doctor to come in.

As it turned out, she was okay, the injury was minor, and my stress was resolved. It's true that most of the time things work out—if not immediately, then eventually. From one point of view, stress is a gift; it helps us survive. Our bodies are wired for it. To experience stress is to be alive. No stress, no life. Due to untold years of life's evolution, we have extraordinary capacity to deal with the worst possible situations. Unless you are in a situation in which you do happen to die—which is rarely the case—the stress resolves, and you find that, once more, you are still here, still alive. There will be a tomorrow.

Most of the magazine and internet articles about meditation emphasize that its goal is to become calmer and more relaxed. That is true, as far as it goes. Becoming calmer is one tangible benefit of meditation. But when I taught meditation, I would say that the deeper purpose of meditation is not to be calm per se, but most of all to be *real*—in other words, to be grounded in the truth of what is happening to you. If you are stressed out, then it is part of your meditation to become fully aware of being stressed out. Don't make a big effort to push it aside, don't try to be some other way. In that moment, being stressed is who you are. Being stressed is deeply true.

The minute you embrace that fact with both arms, you will actually become less stressed and more awake. You will be rooted in what's real *and* hopefully calmer. But whether you are calm or not, your meditation is working. In a real emergency, you don't have time to meditate or to be calm. You just have to be completely present, as I was in the ER for my wife.

I once saw an interview on television with an army commando, a Green Beret. The interviewer said, "It's amazing how you guys can be so free of fear in those incredibly dangerous situations you are in."

The Green Beret replied, "Free of fear? Are you kidding? Do you have any idea what we do? We can be afraid; sometimes we're flat-out terrified. That's all right; fear is what keeps us alive. We don't train to be fearless; we train to accomplish the mission in spite of the fear. The point is to make good decisions, get the job done, and get everyone out alive."

It struck me that this Green Beret understood, in his own way, an important truth about meditation. To be successful, whatever his state of mind, he had to be real. Anything less wouldn't work. The same is true of meditation.

Our second reflection explores the "spiritual" domain. I put the word *spiritual* in quotes because I'm not a big fan of how the word is used these days. Through overuse, it has been bleached of most of its original meaning. Instead of the word *spiritual* I prefer the phrase *big question*, because that is what we are really talking about. When it comes to aging, as well as life in general, there are small questions, medium questions, and big questions. Small questions might be things like diet, exercise, weight loss, medical checkups, and so on. It is relatively easy to make a checklist of the small questions.

Medium questions concern emotional health: stress, worry, and maintaining a sense of well-being. I call these "medium" because they are harder to get a handle on and more challenging to accomplish. Just making a checklist won't suffice. It's more a matter of maintaining a healthy attitude in spite of your regret at goals not met, at past mistakes that cannot be corrected, and at the feeling that your life could have unfolded differently. The best remedy for these kinds of unhappy reflections is to remember what my Buddhist teacher said: "Every breath, new chances." Your life is never over as long as you are breathing. As long as you are alive there can be new beginnings. So, these medium questions are more elusive and challenging, but they do have solutions.

The big questions are big precisely because they don't really have solutions at all; in fact, they are mysteries. What is the meaning of any human life—of your life? What aspects of your life really count, and which ones can you leave behind as you grow older? Why is the world such an unhappy place, generation after generation? What will happen when you die?

Each of the world's religions aims to provide answers to these big questions, and if you are someone who follows a faith-centered life, your faith may offer sustenance. My Buddhist faith sustains me, and I draw comfort and satisfaction from its teachings. Buddhism readily acknowledges the ultimate mystery of existence and the evanescence of a human life. Yet it encourages us to enjoy each moment, each day, each person and object fully, as we don't know when that moment may be our last.

Whatever your faith, even if it is no faith, the important thing is to acknowledge the seminal importance of the big questions. They are perennial. They were there when you were a child, asking your parents where you came from and who made God. As you grew to adulthood, the big questions might have faded into the woodwork of a busy adult life. But when aging comes, the big questions return. Aging sparks the rebirth of the big questions.

The more you age, the more you know that somewhere out there, the end will come—the biggest question of all. It's not something you need to dwell on, but one of the blessings of aging is that it can reconnect you with the two most consequential moments in your life—your birth and your death. There was a moment of mystery when you came into this world, and according to that same mystery, you will one day be gone. To contemplate this magic is to touch something extraordinary.

Our deep reflection begins with the phrase *big question*. Repeat it: *big question, big question*. Each one of us has a big question. It rises and falls on every breath; it knocks on the door of awareness with every heartbeat. Your deep mind already knows all about the big question, and saying the words brings it forward.

You don't say "big question" because you expect an answer. The reason the big question is big is that there is no answer. It abides as a question—the question of your being here at all, or as the physicist Stephen Hawking put it in his version of the big question, "Why is there anything at all?" As you continue your investigation into the big question, let your deep mind find an image, something nonverbal, that expresses this big mysterious feeling. It could be something from nature, like a venerable old tree. It could be a person that you love. It could be your long-gone parents, suddenly reappearing to remind you that it is because of them and their love for each other that you are here.

When I search for an image of the big question, what comes up for me is the sound of a bell being struck. I have the thought that the ringing of a bell is like being born. There was a day in 1947 in a hospital in Southern California when I took my first breath and cried my first cry. That's true for you too, in a different year in a different town.

Your big question, and the image or sound that comes to you along with it, is the crux of your reflection—your meditation on the expansive crucible that holds and maintains your unique spirit. Rest with it, not needing anything else to happen or any answer to come. Bigness itself is a respite from the smallness and occasional weariness of aging. There will come a day when you and I and everyone will return to whence we came and will no longer be here. Until then, let bigness embrace you.

Every person has a part of them that is big. It doesn't matter how your life has gone or whether you feel good about how things are now. You are still big, as big as big can be.

That is big enough.

9

RETIREMENT

We all remember what retirement meant for men when we were growing up. We saw our fathers and our father's friends do it. They worked until they were retirement age: sixty-five, or younger in some professions. They drew on Social Security and maybe a pension. They had ten more years of active healthy life, since life expectancy was in the mid-seventies in those days. They played golf or had hobbies, had a drink or two before dinner, and got together with their retired buddies and talked about sports, politics, and the weather.

At least that was the cultural norm. Today, retirement is not so much a moment in time when you stop going to work. It is now more of a gradual process, if it happens at all. Sometimes it leads to another kind of work—often called an *encore career*. Sometimes retirement doesn't happen at all.

I was getting coffee in Starbuck's one day when I struck up a conversation with an employee on break, a man in his sixties. He introduced himself as Charles. I asked him if he was the manager.

"No," Charles said. "Just a barista." He paused.

I sensed a story in his hesitation. "Do you like the work?"

Charles shrugged. "It doesn't matter. I just need the money. Who can live on Social Security?"

"I see," I said. "What kind of work did you used to do?"

"I sold insurance," Charles said. "The company I worked for downsized, and I took early retirement. Not really a choice."

Charles's Starbucks job was not really an encore career; he had to do it to pay the bills. Charles's situation is all too common. A recent article in Investopedia reported that 45 percent of baby boomers have no retirement savings.[1] Magazines such as AARP's that have popularized the term *encore career* to make it sound exciting, like an encore at the opera. Sometimes that is so, but Charles's Starbucks job was simply a necessity.

According to a recent article by Andrew Soergel, these days one in four Americans *never* plan or expect to retire.[2] The reasons vary, but the most common reason cited was financial. A financial advisor told me that the median net worth of couples fifty-five years old was $110,000—not nearly enough for retirement. These statistics are sobering, particularly since, depending on their profession, older people may not have the physical ability or stamina to continue working to provide for their retirement needs. Injury and illness—not to mention age discrimination—all take their toll.

The good news from Andrew Soergel's report is that three out of four Americans *do* expect to retire, and what happens when they do is in flux. No longer is retirement just golf and hobbies. As life expectancy pushes past eighty—with many older men living healthy and productive lives well past that age—men are looking for something new and engaging to do, something that is more than a hobby and more like a new career. Men yoke their identity to their work, and when they don't have a job to do, they tend to drift—even become depressed. *Encore career* may be the current term of art, but I prefer the term fulfilling work. Fulfilling work is work that you want to do, rather than a paying job that you have to do. Sometimes fulfilling work provides a paycheck just like your former paying job, and sometimes it is more like volunteering. But it is fulfilling and real; it strengthens and preserves a man's sense of identity, a sense of who he is.

Over the last few years, I myself have shifted from my paying job as owner of a software business to the more fulfilling work of writing and music. The software business I founded and ran for thirty-five years is gone now, though at its peak, it had more than thirty corporate clients. That business supported our family through the high-expense years of raising our son and sending him to college. I have already written four books—I began writing books when my software business was still thriving—and this book is my fifth. I am retired from software now, but not from writing. As a writer, I don't ever intend to retire. Writing is in my blood. My avocation as a pianist and composer has been lifelong; that was the career for which I was originally trained but which I never pursued as a livelihood. I'll never give up that part of my life either—it's an old saying that musicians never retire! By being able to shift my focus from paying work to fulfilling work, I consider myself fortunate. Many men never reach that stage and, like Charles, need to continue earning a paycheck however they can.

For me, the shift from work-for-pay to fulfilling work was not a sudden thing. As each software client fell away, my income dropped, and my free time increased. It went on like that, gradually, for several years. The decision to move out of our home was part and parcel of that process, though it began with a much smaller decision just to remodel our downstairs bathroom. Like many two-income professional couples, we had put off major changes to the house, thinking that we would do it when we were older and "had more time." That's a telling phrase—"had more time"—as though time is something we can store in a cellar, like a bottle of wine. "When we were older" is a telling phrase too. It means that we still thought that aging was something yet to happen, not something that was already happening.

But now here we were. My software business was nearly done for, and Amy's career as a teacher and school administrator had ended. She was now a so-called retired teacher, though in terms of her skills she remained a teacher and could teach or tutor again. For us, remodeling the bathroom was a first tentative step toward full retirement, though at first it just seemed like another nice-to-have.

Our contractor came out to take a look at our bathroom. He had some good ideas—floor-to-ceiling tile in the shower, a picture window looking out into our private garden. We asked how much it would cost if we did everything but the window. "Oh, I don't know," he said. "Maybe $15,000 in round numbers."

As the contractor was leaving, I casually mentioned to him how much we loved the house. "Yes," I said, without thinking, "it has lots of stairs, and we are getting older, but I hear stair lifts are getting cheaper and who knows, maybe we'll put in an elevator so we can live here into our nineties."

It wasn't until a few hours later, after dinner, that Amy lapsed into an uncomfortable silence. "What's the matter?" I asked.

She became angry. "You never listen to me!" she exclaimed. "You never ask me anything. I don't want to live in this house until we're ninety!"

I had considered my comments to the contractor just small talk, but obviously I had missed something big. Unbeknownst to me, Amy had been thinking much further into the future than I had. As I indicate in the next chapter, "What Women Know," this dynamic between wives and husbands is not uncommon. The wife privately starts making long-term plans well before the husband.

We quickly realized that our next step was not remodeling the bathroom, it was selling the house. Once we realized that we were facing that major decision, our life changed dramatically. Up to this point, I hadn't thought about retirement per se; I was just going along with my life. Once we dove headfirst into preparing our big house for sale and searching for a smaller one in a quieter, more rural community, I realized that retirement was really a big deal; it meant readying ourselves for the last phase of life. Just uttering the phrase "last phase of life" was daunting, even a little scary. What did that mean? For us it meant finding a house with no stairs, a house in a community full of neighbors who could help us out if we became infirm, a house near a bus route if we could no longer drive, a house where one of us could continue to live alone if the other one was gone. Each of these considerations meant major readjustment. Our life wasn't over, not by any means. But once we completed this move, our old life would be over. Once that bridge was crossed, there would be no going back.

These were indeed serious facts to think about. Making preparations for the gradual decline of our capabilities and, worst of all, the loss of one of us, was not a job I had much enthusiasm about. But we both took it on. As I reflected on the various effects downsizing would have on our life, including our money, I had to came to realize that financially—if for no other reason—we had to move. We had two big mortgages, and—though I didn't like admitting it—with the slow decline in my software income, which had crept up on us, we were now living beyond our means. Our ticket to long-term financial viability lay in the equity in our home, which—since we lived in the San Francisco area—had increased substantially due to the high-tech housing boom. San Francisco now has the dubious distinction of having a higher cost of living than Manhattan. The average rent for a one-bedroom apartment is now over $3,000, a fact that has created a housing and homelessness crisis. But from our point of view as homeowners, it was a good time to sell.

I now became conscious of how much worrying about money had been a background presence in my mind. There had been other times when, as a small-business owner, I faced crises. I've already noted that there were times I wasn't sure I could make payroll or even stay in business. The year I nearly died from encephalitis I was unable to work much for nearly a year, and I had to rely on my employees to carry on as best they could. I dodged all those bullets with a combination of good timing and good luck, but those nagging money worries never left me.

I learned what all of us who are aging need to always remember: unless you are truly wealthy, in preparing for retirement, worrying about money comes with the territory.

Everybody Needs Money

There is a line from the 2001 movie *Heist* that I have always liked. Actor Danny DeVito plays Mickey Bergman, a small-time criminal. At one point, Mickey Bergman says, with a gleam in his eye, "Everybody needs money. That's why they call it money." This David Mamet line is funny in a mordant sort of way, but it's hard to explain why. It's clearly saying something that's true—even profound—but it's hard to put your finger on what that is. When Bergman says, "That's why they call it money," the line reminds us that money is a big deal—particularly for men, but increasingly for women too. In our society, how much money you have goes a long way toward establishing your overall status and value as a human being. It shouldn't be that way, perhaps, but it is.

When I was in the rehab hospital, my family was overjoyed that I wasn't paralyzed, that I could see and hear, that I could talk normally, that my mind seemed whole. I didn't feel that way at all. I felt embarrassed that I was so weak. But most of all I feared that my brain had lost its computer skills, which meant that I wouldn't be able to earn money and that I would be effectively worthless. That wasn't an unfounded fear. Many people with my illness do permanently lose their high-level cognitive skills. As it turned out, my fears were groundless. In time I found that my software skills had been unaffected. Before long I was doing programming on my laptop propped up in my hospital bed. My employees could have done that work, but it was important for me to do it, to prove to myself that I was still capable, that I still had worth, that I was still a man who could earn money and be seen as valuable.

Earlier in my recovery, I had entertained dire fantasies: that we would lose the house, that my wife would lose respect for me and leave me, that I would end up alone, living in a leaky trailer in an RV park, or worse. These were the night terrors of a man who didn't know if he was still a man, who didn't know if his core identity was still intact, who didn't know if he could still have a life.

Yes, money is a big deal. Everywhere you look there are books, articles, websites, and podcasts about retirement finances, investments, budgeting—all the external logistics of managing this major concern of the retirement years. But few of these resources discuss the inner aspect of money worries—the stress, the uncertainty, the looming specter of going broke by living too long (which otherwise ought to be a good thing) and dying in poverty.

I remember something the *San Francisco Chronicle*'s John Wasserman once wrote about wealthy people: "There is nothing so relaxed as the shoulders of a wealthy person when the talk turns to money." Wasserman imagined a scenario where a group of people—one of whom is extremely rich—are working out how to divvy up the check after lunch at a restaurant. The rich person dutifully puts in his share for a sandwich and salad, while his friends all quietly realize that he could buy the restaurant one hundred times over and barely notice it in his bank account. If you are one of these uber-wealthy people, more power to you! But, chances are, you are not, and like most people, worries about money take up a lot more of your mental time and resources than you would like.

Part of what retirement means is that you have less earning power—sometimes much less—than at your peak. Not only do you earn less, but you are likely past the point in life when you can, through a new job or career, increase or regenerate your earning power. You have Social Security, possibly a pension, hopefully a nest egg that generates a monthly draw, and that is that. As any financial advisor can tell you, the most pertinent question once you have reached this stage is whether you have enough money to last until you die. These days, the investment industry runs those numbers out to age ninety-five, as Jim, my own financial adviser, informed me.

I remember the first time he told us that he was going to calculate our lifetime need for money based on a life expectancy of ninety-five. "Whoa!" I said. "We're not going to live to be ninety-five. I'm not sure I want to live to be ninety-five."

"You might not live to ninety-five," Jim replied. "But suppose you do. People are living longer and longer. I have other clients who are in their nineties, who are mentally alert and physically healthy. You have to plan for that possibility. Ninety-five is the new standard in financial planning."

I have already mentioned that the median retirement savings for baby boomers in 2019 was $110,000—a too-small number for millions of savings-challenged people. If you are one of those people, you can read on the internet, in *AARP* magazine, and in myriad other resources what you might do about that. But few of these resources discuss how it *feels* not to have enough for retirement—particularly how it feels for men. Our generation of men were socialized to see ourselves as primary breadwinners. That role may also be hardwired into our DNA as hunters who brought home the meat. Whatever the reason, the ability to earn is closely tied to our inner sense of status, worth, and core identity.

How else to explain the men who jumped out of windows or who otherwise ended their lives when the Great Depression put 30 percent of them out of work? There is no logic to such a drastic act. An unemployed but living man is certainly far more valuable to his family than a dead one. But men did choose ultimate self-destruction rather than face the extreme sense of worthlessness that not having money induced.

Kinds of Retirement

These days, there is no one kind of retirement. Broadly speaking, I can identify four different types. First there is traditional retirement, in which you stop working completely, live off your savings, and enjoy a life free from work. For some people, this can include traveling to all those places in the world you dreamed of visiting and never had the time or money to visit. For others it is enhancing the home—remodeling the kitchen, collecting wine, building a woodshop in the garage. The key requirement for traditional retirement is money. If you have the money, you can do what you want.

One cautionary point: remember the old canard, "Money can't buy happiness"? Well, it really can't. These days there are dot-com millionaires who can afford to retire when they are thirty. They have the resources to live the life of their dreams, but the question is: are those dreams truly satisfying, or do they simply paper over a deeper dissatisfaction?

The second flavor of retirement is what I have already termed *fulfilling work*. This is work that gives you deep satisfaction, whether or not it pays you a penny. Sometimes this takes the form of volunteering. I once met a man named Rich who had made a good living as a financial manager. Now retired, he volunteered his expertise managing the finances of a crisis clinic for abused women.

"I'm doing a lot of the same things that I used to be paid big bucks for," Rich told me. "But I'm enjoying it a hell of a lot more."

Another form of fulfilling work is pursuing a long-deferred avocation or talent that you never had the time for when you were fully employed. My passion for music is an example of this. My parents had imagined a career for me as a professional musician. They had even picked out in their minds the pianist in Paris they wanted me to study with. Unfortunately for their dreams, I figured out two things by the time I was twenty. First, I wasn't good enough for the big time; and second, a successful musician's life means constant travel, and I hated to travel. Instead, I have kept the musical flame alive throughout my years of full-time employment, and now I have the time and resources to devote much more time to it than before. You may have a talent or avocation like that. If you do, and you can afford to do it, by all means plan to devote yourself to it as soon as you can. Whether it's volunteering or avocation, fulfilling work is not really retirement as much as reinvention.

The third kind of retirement is no retirement at all—that is, you just keep working. As I mentioned, 25 percent of the population—and probably a higher percentage of men—don't plan to ever retire. This may be due to financial necessity, or it may be like the lawyer recently featured in the news who, at ninety-nine, still went to the office every morning, still saw clients, and was still sharp as a tack.[3] My own personal physician just turned seventy-five. He kept telling his patients he was going to retire, but last I checked in with him he's postponed it yet again. "I enjoy what I'm doing too much," he said.

In the case of the ninety-nine-year-old lawyer or my physician, perhaps we could say that for them, career and fulfilling work are one and the same. If you have the good luck to be like them, then your no-retirement plans are already made. Just keep doing what you are doing.

The fourth kind of retirement is the non-retirement of Charles the Starbucks barista. He had to keep working because he couldn't afford not to. Regrettably many baby boomers now find themselves in this situation, and there is not much that can be done, except to watch your costs like a hawk and, if absolutely necessary, relocate where the cost of living is cheaper. At the very least, if you aren't already on Medicare, try to find employment with health benefits. And take care of your health so that you have the energy and wherewithal to keep working.

In the fifty-five-plus village we now live in, the people we have met in our daily walks and at social events represent all these different categories. Fifty-five is not so old, so some of the residents are still working full-time. I see them driving off in their cars early in the morning as in any other neighborhood.

We've also met some who are semiretired and now work out of a home office part time. Among them are a lawyer, an accountant, writers and editors, tutors, real estate brokers, a jazz drummer, and several psychotherapists. Of those still working, I don't know how many are still doing it for the money, but I would venture most are pursuing their vision of fulfilling work and enjoying the continuation of their profession and expertise.

There are also a number of older women living alone, as well as some men. Some of them are widows or widowers, some divorcees. Regrettably, a large percentage of older people—by the time they are eighty, it is nearly 40 percent, according to the U.S. Census—do live alone. It's hard to live alone—hard for men particularly.

Deep Mind Reflection: Retirement

I suggest two keywords for this reflection: *retirement* and *retire*. One is a noun, the other a verb, and each word offers a different flavor. *Retirement* is a stage of life, or a stage of work and career, that you are in. *Retire* is the active intention. I suggest that if you are not yet retired that you try using *retire* rather than *retirement*. It can be internally spoken as a kind of question: *Retire?*

You can imagine yourself looking in the mirror and having your mirror image ask you: Okay, my friend. Retire? Soon? Later? Never? Have you even started thinking about it?

If you are already retired, or close to it, you could try the key-word *retirement*. That too could come up as a question: Retirement? How do I feel about it? How is it going? Am I happy? Sad? At loose ends? Not sure what to do?

When you have honed in on the appropriate keyword, see what image floats into awareness. Your deep mind undoubtedly has one for you. The image that comes to mind might surprise you. It might express a different emotion than the one you imagine you are feeling.

For example, you may be searching the web for exciting vacation spots or foreign cities to visit—creating what people these days call a bucket list (which, of course, may be vastly altered now since the pandemic). However, your deep mind might bring up an image of your children or grandchildren, who, if you thought about it, might love to see more of you.

When I do this reflection, I use the keyword *retirement*, because the word retired doesn't fit where I think I am. I don't think I'm retired. In fact, I am working on several projects—such as this book! Writing a book is a three-year marathon, and it's hard work. After you write, you have to promote, you have to speak, you have to travel. I'm just hoping that at my age I still have the stamina for it.

The image that comes to my mind when I think of retirement is a picture of the tall blue spruce that grows in the back yard of our new house. It's been there a long time, and it stands with dignity and poise. It's probably survived more than forty winters, and at this point, it would take a lot to push it over.

I suppose my deep mind is coming up with that image because it wants me to think of myself like that. I remember Erikson's ego identity—what I renamed deep acceptance—and I ask myself, Have I arrived there? Do I have deep acceptance about my life? I think deep acceptance is an important feature of a good retirement. In fact, that may be the last, and perhaps the most important, meaning of retirement: stepping back and retiring from striving to be better, higher, richer, more accomplished, more famous, and simply resting in what you have done and who you have become.

I'm glad I have the blue spruce to remind me of this.

10

WHAT WOMEN KNOW

To the male readers of this book who are married to or in partnership with a woman, I have news for you: the woman in your life is one of the best sources of good information about your own aging. This is true for two reasons. First, your partner knows you better than anyone. She listens to what you say (and don't say) day in and day out. Second, women, in general, are more tuned in to their own aging bodies than men are to theirs. Their sensitivity makes them tuned in to your aging too.

This chapter is designed to send two simple messages: one to you and one to your partner. Message to you: you need to know what she knows. You may think you already know, but, chances are, you don't fully know—or even if you do, you could still probably know more. Message to your partner: I hope in this chapter to give some tools and suggestions about how to better communicate what you know to your husband or partner.

While it's true that older couples grow old together, how well they share and communicate their aging experience varies a lot. Marriage counselors will tell you that for younger couples, the most frequent culprits for conflict are sex and money. For older couples, a third culprit enters the picture—sometimes openly, sometimes stealthily—the shadow of aging.

I have mentioned that the majority of the readers of my book *Aging as a Spiritual Practice* are women. At workshops they often say, "I tried to get my husband to come, but he wouldn't. He just said, 'Tell me if you learn anything interesting.'" Most men don't like to talk about aging, particularly in public or in front of their wives. Women's willingness to share their husbands' issues gives them a coping resource that men lack.

In other words, a couple's experiences of aging are often not aligned—particularly when there is a significant age difference between them. The woman knows what her husband is thinking, and when she gets together with her friends, they talk about their husbands' aging issues.

This chapter presents—through interviews and anecdotes—what women actually think and feel about the men they love and care about. I hope to help women communicate this knowledge to the men in their lives. I also hope that women reading this chapter will feel supported and validated in knowing that their experience is similar to other women's experiences.

Health professionals I have talked with generally concur that women are more realistic about aging and more willing than men to share their experiences of aging with each other. When women get together to talk—and older women do this often, sometimes one-on-one, but often in small groups of friends—their own aging is a common topic. The aging issues of the men in their lives is another common topic, but what they talk about among themselves typically stays confidential. Men aren't at the table when these discussions take place, and women aren't likely to rush home and tell their partner or spouse that he was a key topic of conversation among their friends.

In short, there is a divide between men and women when it comes to aging. Some of this divide might be accounted for by studies showing that when women talk to each other they experience a rise in oxytocin levels—oxytocin being the "feel-good" hormone that accounts for various instances of elevated mood, including the so-called runner's high.[1] Men don't experience this conversational mood lift when they talk among themselves. So women enjoy talking among themselves, regardless of the topic.

Another possible reason why men are less attuned to their own aging is that they don't have the same variation in their body experiences that women do. Starting with puberty, continuing with each monthly period, along with pregnancy and menopause, women regularly experience changes in their bodies. The bodily changes of aging—and menopause is just one example—are front and center for women in a way they are not for men. This means that men can imagine—or, in some cases, fool themselves into thinking—that aging isn't really happening to them and that they can, physically and mentally, do most of what they could do when they were twenty or even thirty years younger. Just among my circle of men friends, I know four who sustained serious injuries while bicycling with a group of much younger men—injuries that included a broken hand, broken collarbone, serious concussion, and, in one case, a fractured skull. My small sample is not a generalized proof of this phenomenon, so consult your own experience and those of your own friends to see if this proposal has merit. We men, in assessing our physical strength and capacity, tend to mentally subtract years from our biological age. On the other hand, women undoubtedly spend more on ways to look younger than men do. That is because a woman's physical appearance is more central to their attractiveness and desirability than it is for men.

Kate

Kate was a professional woman in her sixties. Kate told me she got together once a week with a group of four or five friends to have lunch and chat. Kate and two others of the group were still working, and the other two had only recently retired, so they talked through what it was like to maintain a professional career at their age, how their male bosses regularly looked past them in meetings and work assignments in favor of younger women, and how hard it was to keep going when you needed a nap after lunch and there was no time or place to have one.

They also talked about their own health issues. One of them had recently had a knee replacement; another was thinking about a hip replacement. They were all past menopause but still had occasional hot flashes and other distressing symptoms like migraines that their doctors told them were medically insignificant—though that didn't help with the difficulty they caused.

Three of the women were married; two were divorced. Kate said that at some point, usually just before dessert, the talk would turn to their husbands—or ex-husbands—and their marital frustrations. "He still wants sex twice a week, like clockwork," said one woman, "and I'm really and truly not that interested. Sometimes he jokes that maybe he'll have to find a younger woman. I really don't get that joke—not at all."

"I should be so lucky," Marilyn responded. "Cliff has completely lost interest—to the point that he barely remembers to kiss me before he turns over and goes to sleep. I know he's worried that he can't perform, but that's a lot more important to him than it is to me. Whatever the reason, he doesn't have to shut me out like I'm half dead."

"He should go to the doctor," Kate replied. "They have all kinds of ways now—not just pills."

"He doesn't like his doctor," Marilyn said, "He thinks he scolds too much. At least last year he went for his physical, but he didn't like hearing he had to stop smoking and lose twenty pounds. I've tried to cut down on the red meat, but he gets mad if he doesn't have his steak medium-rare every Saturday night. Old habits die hard."

Joanne

Joanne, a psychologist with extensive experience in group counseling and facilitation, confirmed my sense of the communication issues about aging between women and their husbands.

"Yes, I see this both in my individual therapy clients and in my women's groups," Joanne said to me. "Aging is a topic that couples often have difficulty talking about. Women usually have a better sense of what is really going on with their husbands than their husbands themselves do. They can't talk about it with their husbands, so they come here and talk about it in my groups."

Another of Joanne's clients could see that her husband was not exercising as much as his cardiologist had told him to, and he became dizzy when he didn't drink enough water—another directive from a doctor that he wasn't following.

"My clients have lots of stories like that," Joanne concluded. "Here's another: a woman client came to me rather upset and reported that she and her husband's sex life was not going well. Recently he had found difficulty maintaining an erection, even sometimes with an erectile dysfunction pill, and this bothered him to no end. My client said that she told her husband repeatedly that this was not a pressing issue for her. They had had a satisfying sex life with good communication for most of their marriage. 'At this point, it doesn't matter that much whether the pill works or not,' she said. 'The important thing for me is that we are close, that we still have intimacy. There are ways you can satisfy me other than regular intercourse.'

"Well," said Joanne, "That just seemed to make things worse for this client. 'Well, it may not matter to you,' her husband said, 'but it sure as hell matters to me. I thought these pills were supposed to take care of the problem. I don't want to be half a man. I want things to be the way they used to be.'"

Joanne told her client that it seemed to her that this issue was operating on several levels and that sexual satisfaction for either her husband or for her may not be the most important. "It sounds to me like the core problem is that your husband sees his sexual performance as a reflection of his competence as a person and his worth in your eyes. This is not something you are going to be able to talk him out of. The two of you probably need some couples' counseling, if he'd be willing to go. In the meantime, he should probably check with his doctor. There are other remedies for erectile dysfunction besides Viagra."

Eileen

Eileen's husband, Terry, after a serious heart attack, had a pacemaker installed. The doctors told him that the pacemaker would help control his heart rhythm, but he was still at risk of another heart attack. He had to take medicine at regularly spaced intervals throughout the day and periodically wear a monitor to measure his heart's performance.

"It's hard on both of us, worrying about that," Eileen said. "Of course, it's hard on him. He's the one who is ill and who has to be vigilant all the time. But it's hard on me too. He doesn't like having me hover. I get that, if I were him, I would feel the same way. But if he faints, he can fall, and if he falls, he can break a leg or hit his head. That hasn't happened yet, but I worry about it every day."

I asked Eileen to think of one thing she wanted to say to her husband but didn't feel she could.

"I want to say to him, 'let me help you,'" Eileen said. "'I love you, and all I want to do is make sure you don't get hurt.' But he has his pride. He doesn't want to feel that somebody else needs to take care of him."

I asked Eileen if she had other concerns.

"I worry that something will happen when I'm not there," Eileen said. "He feels safe when he's in the house, so that's where he likes to be." She paused. "My worst nightmare is that he'll have a heart attack when he's here alone, and I won't be here for him. That's the scenario that keeps me up nights."

Rachel

Rachel was a retired psychotherapist who had been married to the same man for nearly forty years. I thought that the combination of her personal and professional experience would prove to be a fruitful resource in discussing women's insights about men aging. I started by describing to her my sense that there was a heroic aspect in men's facing their own aging as the last and often biggest challenge of their lives.

"Yes," Rachel said, "but I think there is also an aspect of surrender that is quite important. My older male clients often begin their work with me with an emphasis on doing, on competence, on strength. I work with them to help them set those aspects aside and surrender into an area where competence and strength aren't effective.

"Many times, these clients present with some problem in their marriage, some longstanding issue that has only been exacerbated with time and age.

"You know," she continued, "I think that as men age, and their testosterone decreases, they often get sweeter. That's a real opportunity for couples to find a different quality of partnership, with more willingness to communicate. There are changes in a man's body and soul as he ages that can affect a marriage profoundly."

"What role can a wife or partner play in encouraging that change?" I asked.

"On the whole, women are more relational than men," Rachel replied. "When they look at their aging husband, they don't just look at his problems or issues in isolation. They look at how those things affect the whole relationship."

"Can you give my women readers any suggestions or advice on how to support their partners as they face aging's changes?"

"Well," Rachel said, "as the need to be competent and strong falls away in a man, a new kind of energy starts to get freed up. There's the opportunity for learning, for a spiritual and artistic self to emerge. It's a shift away from doing and more asking, 'What is my soul saying to me?' That's the heart of it: let go of the death grip of who you used to be. Women need to watch for those changes in a man and quietly encourage them. They can do it. Women are very observant, very tuned in, in a relationship. They see these things.

"It's funny," Rachel continued, "men think that women want them to be strong. But that's not how it is, usually. Most women welcome vulnerability in a man. They long for it."

I asked Rachel to shift her focus to her personal experiences in her own marriage.

"That's how it's been for us," Rachel replied. "In the last few months my husband has been dealing with severe back pain. It's made him quite vulnerable. He hasn't been able to do things he used to always be able to do. I've had to do the lifting, the carrying, the putting things away. And it's brought us closer, that role reversal."

"Yes," I said, "My wife and I had the same experience during the times I was ill. At first, I didn't like it at all, but eventually I was just so grateful that she was able to do all those things, even pay the bills, stuff I always used to do."

"Right," Rachel said. "And one final thing that both men and women need to remember is the importance of laughter. You have to have a sense of humor when disaster strikes, whether it's small or large. You know—just take delight in the small things, like being able to eat ice cream together. You can take life so seriously when you get old. There's a quality of lovely absurdity to it, the way you can't really manage or control anything.

"Laughter," Rachel concluded, "is the greatest surrender of all."

Kelly

Kelly was a professional woman of sixty-six, still working, as was her husband. Kelly, like many of the women I interviewed, met for lunch regularly with a group of women friends, and she confirmed that one of the regular topics of conversation was their aging husbands.

"My friends tell me that while they are already thinking about aging and retirement—often three, five, or more years down the road—their husbands can't seem to visualize what comes next. I think it's because women are trained and socialized to be multitaskers. We track kids and shopping and work and social engagements all at once, all the time.

"On the other hand, two of my friends have husbands who have recently retired, and it seems like they're really depressed about the loss of job identity."

Kelly also felt that when it comes to physically taking care of one's body, women do better than men. When men start having their aches and pains, Kelly said, only then do they start looking around for remedies; but women have been doing that for a long time. "Suddenly the men start shuffling around, feeling like they're an old man," Kelly said. "Women have decades of experience not feeling well sometimes. We don't buckle that easily."

Kelly's circle of women friends all seemed to wish that they could communicate better with their husbands about all of this. "Retired men suddenly have all this time on their hands," she said. "You think they'd want to spend some of that time talking, but it doesn't seem to work that way."

In addition to communicating, Kelly and her friends wanted to work on different ways for them and their husbands to show and express affection for each other. "Sex doesn't have to be like it was when we were thirty. It doesn't even have to be sex. What about just touching or hugging?"

When I asked Kelly to sum up what she and her friends felt was most important, Kelly said, "In a way, getting old is like starting all over again, finding new ways to talk, to do things together, to be loving together. It could be a great adventure!"

Evelyn

"My husband and I live out in the country. It's wonderful. We're surrounded by woods and walking trails and friendly neighbors who are not too close but not too far if we need something. We're both reasonably healthy. My husband's been retired for three years, I just retired from my job as a nurse.

"So in some ways we're living in paradise, the way we always wanted to live. But I look ahead three, five, or ten years, and I wonder what life will be like then. We're in our early seventies now, but in ten years, we'll be in our early eighties. What will life be like then?"

"Do you and your husband talk about it?" I asked.

"No," Evelyn said, "that's the problem. He doesn't want to talk about it. 'Why worry about how we'll be then?' he says. 'Things are great now. Let's just enjoy the life we have and deal with the future in the future.'

"I just can't live that way," Evelyn concluded. "I've always planned ahead. That's how I've always lived my life. I've always been the planner, and he's always been the spontaneous one. That worked really well when we were young, but now I'm not so sure." She sighed. "I wish there were some way I could talk about it with him. I've certainly tried."

How to Talk to Your Husband

Joanne, the therapist, helps women in her groups develop skills to talk to their husbands about health-related issues. "Men typically don't like to be told what to do, especially by their wives," Joanne explained. "On the other hand, wives know their husbands better than anyone else and observe their husbands' behavior day in and day out."

I asked Joanne what were the two or three techniques that she found were most effective for women in speaking to their husbands.

"It depends on the couple, but usually humor is effective," Joanne replied, echoing what Rachel had said. "The woman who was concerned about her husband eating too much bacon found a cute little statue of a pig in a thrift store and put it on the counter next to the stove. A woman sharing concerns about her own health, rather than her husband's, is another effective way to initiate honest conversation. Scientific information—such as an article about diet in a magazine—is usually not as effective."

Deep Mind Reflections

I hope and anticipate that both men and women will read this chapter. To that end, I have provided two reflections: one for men, one for women. Let's begin with the one for women, since that can deepen what you as women already know. If any women readers have skipped ahead in the book to this chapter, I encourage you to read chapter 2, "Guide to Deep Mind Reflection." That will give you a context and overview for this exercise.

For this reflection, I'd like to reverse the usual order and begin with an image. Once you have settled yourself quietly and cleared your mind of all extraneous thoughts and distractions, I encourage you to bring into your mind's eye an image of your aging husband or partner. It can be a picture of his face, which you have come to know so well. It could be his face as he is today, or it could be a picture of him as a younger man, when you first met and fell in love with him, perhaps. In that case, imagine his face changing and growing older year by year until your picture of him settles into the face he has today. You can also provide scenery for this inner video. Perhaps the two of you are sitting at the kitchen table, as you do so often, and you are looking at his face as you actually do every day.

However you construct this visualization, keep in mind the purpose of it—to fill your mind with a vivid image of an older man, a man you know and love.

Once you have settled on this image and firmed it up, allow your deep mind to suggest a word or phrase. It could be something that you would like to tell him but feel you cannot. It could also be something you have told him and which he has either not heard or absorbed, or actively objected to.

I'll give you an example. I'm prediabetic, and I'm constantly struggling to control my weight, which includes restricting my fat intake. One morning I was making a soft-boiled egg.

My wife said, "Do you think you should be having that? It's your third this week."

Without thinking, I snapped back at her, "I can eat an egg if I want!"

I could see from her face that she was upset with me.

That's when I realized how worried she was about my health, how much she wanted to help me, and how resistant I was to accepting her help.

If my wife were doing this deep mind reflection just as you are now, I would encourage her to bring to mind this tense interchange, but in the quietude of her own inner remembering. She could play it out inwardly as though she were replaying a film clip and just watching it.

I have interviewed many women who have played out a similar dynamic with their husbands and have become frustrated or even given up in the face of their husband's resistance.

As you conclude this short reflection, I would ask you to come up with one word or phrase, one that you could hold close as a resource to encourage yourself. It could be a simple word like *patience.* Another possibility would be the phrase *keep trying.* Don't force it. If no word comes, that's all right. But if you are patient and listening to your inner voice closely, your deep mind might offer you some new language and a fresh approach to what might seem to be a chronic problem.

Your husband is probably just like I was, when I heard my wife question me about the egg. I had a reactive response, but underneath, I realized that she was only doing it because she loved me.

Love is what this exercise and reflection is all about.

The second reflection is for male readers. Having read this chapter, by now you have realized—if you hadn't before—that the woman in your life is full of complex and nuanced observations about you as an aging man. Perhaps you have already begun to reflect on the possibility that, however well you know each other and however long you have been together, there are aspects of your relationship and communication that can now go deeper as you age together.

You may want to sit down with her and simply ask, "Do you have concerns about my aging that you would like to share with me but haven't? Have you tried, and have I turned you aside or shut you off without being aware of it?"

That would certainly be a worthy and valuable conversation. But in preparation for that, I suggest that you first follow along with this brief deep mind reflection. Settle yourself quietly as usual, and clear your mind of all extraneous thoughts and concerns. Tune in, as though to a radio channel, to a voice—a woman's voice—and imagine that it is trying to tell you something. See if you can make out what it is.

This is an exercise of receptive imagination, so don't try to anticipate or influence what the message will be. For the moment, don't personalize the voice; don't think of it as your partner's voice. Rather, imagine it as a voice from the ether, from the sky. In fact, it is a voice from your own deep mind. When you can make out the words, repeat them to yourself and make them your own.

When I do this exercise, the words I hear—once I can make out the words—are "don't be proud." I don't think of myself as proud—most proud people don't. But I suppose I am; that is what my inner voice is telling me. I am proud of my life accomplishments and my masteries—which, I realize, may indeed be obscuring from me a simpler truth which my wife can so clearly see. Yes, those masteries are real, but they are or will soon be diminishing, and my aging body is already showing the signs. The person who loves me most in the world can clearly see that—and could tell me, if I were inclined to listen.

Your ethereal voice likely will tell you something different, but whatever it is, note it and accept it. As you do, let your deep mind come up with a picture that expresses what the voice has said. These pictures you imagine in these deep mind reflections are more powerful than any words. Before human beings had language, they had dreams, and dreams speak in the language of images.

This picture could be of your partner, your spouse who loves you and wishes to speak more clearly to you. It could be of something else. Linger on the picture, and see if it changes. It may be trying to tell you a story, one that your partner has been trying to tell you piece by piece.

The picture that comes to me is of a king on a throne—which I suppose represents myself in my pride and my exaggerated, kingly sense of power to stave off the inevitability of my impending decline. And at my side, like a bit player in a Shakespearean drama, is a court jester, gently chiding me for my illusions. I know that this court jester is the one person who can tell the king—me!—anything, because he loves the king. Because the king knows this, he will listen to what the jester says.

Then I understand that the court jester represents my wife. Like the jester, she is the one who loves me and can tell me anything, and I will listen.

This is my deep mind reflection.

Let your own reflection and succession of images morph and change until you feel satisfied that deep mind has conveyed to you what it needs to say. And lastly, let it fade away until it is gone, and you can, as you continue to rest quietly, feel the subtle change it has wrought in your body and spirit.

11

FINAL THOUGHTS

In the writing of this book, I have intermingled my own experiences with those of many others I have spoken to, as well as general thoughts and research results about how men age, gleaned from news articles, therapists, men's group leaders, and other experts in the field. I have included my own story for two reasons. First, it is always better, with any kind of writing, to write about what you know. I'm well versed in my particular saga as an aging man, and whether my experience is like yours, or whether you can relate to the general tenor of my experience, some part of my story is not just unique to me; it applies to many men.

Second, I wanted to share with you how I dealt with my own vulnerabilities and fears. Like most men, I don't like to reveal those things. When I was writing *Healing Lazarus*, my memoir of my near-death and recovery from encephalitis, just before the book was going into production, I suddenly got cold feet. I called up my editor and said, "I can't publish this. I've revealed too many personal secrets. It's all too humiliating. I have to take out a bunch of stuff."

My editor replied, "All those personal secrets are exactly why we are publishing the book. Without that, the book won't be nearly as interesting to your readers."

It's the same with this book. Some part of me would rather not have admitted to the situations that scared me and made me feel that I couldn't cope. But I don't think a book like that would be nearly as compelling or as useful. Remember the lesson of the hospital chaplain, Rev. Hanson: *vulnerability is strength.* That's a lesson we have to keep learning. If you put your dukes up and try to tough it out, the effort makes you rigid, and any stiff wind will push you over. But bend like the willow and let your tears flow, and you'll spring back up, ready for whatever comes next on aging's twisty path.

How Things Turned Out for Me

I have already told our story: for a few months my wife and I were vagabonds, moving from pillar to post, wondering when we would ever land. Fortunately, our journey had a happy ending. In time, we found a smaller house that's just right for us. As I write, we've just celebrated our six-month anniversary in the new house. The boxes are unpacked, the furniture is all in, and the art is on the walls. My beloved piano is in an alcove off the living room. The familiar treasures of a lifetime surround us again. We are home.

Of course, many of our possessions are no longer with us. Goodwill and the Salvation Army are the richer for it. We walk every morning along the wooded walking paths that start a few steps from our front door. We are in farm country now, surrounded on all sides by planted fields that stretch off into the distance and up into the foothills. Sometimes, driving by, we see sheep grazing on the hillside. It wasn't our goal to be in this particular place. But here is where fate and good fortune had us land.

We understand—and accept—that this is likely to be our last house. In all likelihood, one of us will die here. A lot of hard work and good luck has resulted in our being here. Yet it's sobering to think of the words "last house."

Last House

I don't know where you are in your own aging adventure. You may just be starting to think about it, or you may be in your own last house. Some of my friends, hearing about the path we have taken, tell me, "Well, we're going to age in place. We like our house." When I point out to them that they too have stairs and a steep driveway, where a broken ankle or hip replacement would represent an existential crisis, they reply, "We'll deal with that if it happens. For now, we're okay."

Out of politeness, I don't mention what we came to realize: that if we had waited even a couple of years more to make our move, we wouldn't have had the energy to do it. One of aging's imperatives is that, for these big life decisions, you must strike while the iron is hot. We came to recognize that for us, the iron indeed was hot, and we acted with alacrity.

Our ostensible reason for moving was financial (reduce our monthly cost of living) and health-related (preserving our knees by leaving a house with forty stairs), but the deeper reason was to situate ourselves for the long slow glide down to life's end. The fact that as we were doing all this, my sister was living out the last few months of her life, made this point that much more poignant. Making the four-hour drive to sit with her, reminiscing about our whole life together and then driving back in winter rain to resume the daily slog of writing big checks to contractors and enduring the daily mini-crises was a grief-tinged backdrop for this major life change.

I had never imagined I would be at this point in my life. None of us realize that we are growing old or have become old, until we just wake up one morning and see that it is so. This sudden fact is one more measure of declining strength, loss of possibility, loss of virility, loss of a sense of gaining and novelty, and just plain loss.

Yes, aging is loss. It is also a time to be venerable, which is a more elevated term than old. It is true that I am more venerable in some ways. I have a legacy of accomplishment as an author with a modest readership, favorable reviews, and a certain middling acclaim. It is also true that as a writer, you are only as good as your last book, which in my case was seven years ago. The invitations to speak at conferences have dwindled and vanished, the fan letters I used to get with some regularity have dropped way off, the number of literary friends who used to stay in touch regularly is not what it once was.

If I were to measure my stature and standing in the world by such things, I would have to say that I am dwindling, becoming smaller, less visible, less consequential. But as a lifelong Buddhist, steeped in the worldview of that legacy of knowledge and belief, I realize that this state of affairs is written into the fabric of the universe. I am living the teaching that the Buddha taught. All things fade and pass away, including all that we cherish and love—like my sister—including the somewhat glorified images that the ego projects on itself, including our physical body, which actually performs miraculously decade after decade with hardly any attention from us.

Remembering all this—with some gratitude for this Buddhist wisdom that I encountered and internalized when I was young— makes me realize that as the outward shadow of my future life grows shorter, the inward light of what it all means grows longer and more beautiful. There is, indeed, a beauty to all of this—the inevitability of it; the slow, quiet dignity of it; the sense that this is the day-by-day and month-by-month reward for the original gift of life, whose first moments I don't remember, but whose many present moments I eagerly cherish.

Still here, still healthy, still with enough mental horsepower to organize and track the myriad responsibilities of selling a house and buying a house. I can still pull out my laptop and dive back into the elaborate software product I wrote when I was much younger; I can still manage—most of the time—to call up the right word or phrase to write a cogent sentence and paragraph.

Eventually these strengths too will go, and inevitably my mental powers will slow. Until then, I can still learn, still contribute.

Just because I am in my last house doesn't mean it is not an enjoyable and useful house. May it be so for you too, when the time comes.

Discovering Your Essential Household

One thing I discovered in this grand transition is that there is such a thing as an essential household—yet another aspect of inner retirement. From the time we leave home to go to college, move to another town, or rent a first apartment, we establish an essential household. At first it is minimal—a couple of suitcases, a few pieces of furniture, a stuffed bear left over from childhood. But over a lifetime of living in ever larger quarters, earning ever more money, and accumulating ever more possessions, we can forget that we started adult life with a few suitcases of stuff.

"Naked I came from my mother's womb, and naked I shall return," says Job in one of the most frequently quoted passages in the Bible. Job goes on to say, "The Lord giveth, and the Lord taketh away. Blessed be the name of the Lord."

This passage poetically encapsulates the arc of every human life. At the moment of birth, we start with nothing but our own nearly helpless human body. And at the end of life we are in practically the same situation. Everything that we have done, all that we have accumulated, all the people we have known and loved will disappear in a moment. *Aging* is another name for this arc of life. We don't call it *aging* until later in life, but in fact, aging begins when life begins. This short window of time—though life expectancy for men is now approaching eighty in the United States—is the be all and end all of who we are.

Until we leave home at the end of adolescence, we don't have our own essential household; we abide in the household of our parents.

But once we pack our bags and sally forth, we pull together the original contents of this essential package. It grows and expands as we grow and expand. And as Amy and I discovered when, having decided to sell our house and move, after fifty years of steady accumulation—which, in my case, included a garage and attic full of cartons of hard-cover versions of the books I had written—the mountain of stuff we had to go through was overwhelming. Whatever nugget of essential possessions we had started with when we married in our senior year of college and set out to drive across the country with all of it packed in a small trailer behind our car was hidden and invisible deep inside that mountain. It would take us many months to sort through it all. We made make endless trips to the local library to divest ourselves of books we no longer wanted or needed, similarly endless trips to the local Goodwill, and we had a visit from the Salvation Army truck to haul away my mother's vintage California Mission dining-room set that now was too big and out of style and had no resale value.

What I came to realize as the physical shape of our essential household began to emerge from our mountain of possessions is that these core belongings also form an internal structure, a mental placeholder for identity and ego. Our essential household is a deeply buried and mostly unconscious emblem of who we are, who we have always been. Because I am a high-tech professional and software developer, as well as a writer and musician, my smartphone and laptop are at the center of this essential identity. Centuries ago, people towed their essential household behind a horse. These days, we cart our electronic gear from spot to spot, all of it a repository for the digital data that defines our history, our friendships, and our life.

This is the way it will be for all of us now, I imagine. When our last illness comes, when we are fading from life, our essential household will shrink to this. In the last weeks of my sister's life, she was bedridden. She could not stand, dress herself, even walk to the bathroom. Her lifelong love of colorful clothes—always a core element of her identity—had fallen away. She shifted between two dressing gowns, confined to bed day and night. What she still had—and what she still used to maintain her connections and her hold on life—was her iPhone, with photographs of her grandchildren, names and addresses of all her friends, and links to news sites when television news became too distressing and stimulating for her.

So it is now. In ancient times a man on his deathbed would call for his sword, the emblem of his masculinity and identity as a warrior. Or his boots; we still say a man "died with his boots on." These days the last vestige of essential household, core identity, and living presence might be our smartphone, into which, if we wish, we can dictate our last wishes and final messages of love.

So when my wife and I watched our whole household of furniture, art, books, file cabinets full of files, and other nonessential stuff get efficiently packed up and loaded into the mover's van to disappear into storage, what was left? What was the essential household that we loaded into our cars as we trundled off to that noisy extended-stay motel?

I discovered that as our core possessions dwindled down to a couple of carloads, the security of my laptop began to take on outsized importance. Like most software professionals, I have backups everywhere—on other laptops and backup hard drives, some stored in offsite storage, some in safe deposit boxes. But the one laptop I was taking with me to an anonymous motel room had all my latest stuff; it was my prime working space. It had become *me*. I couldn't lose it; if I lost the laptop, I would lose me. How would I secure the laptop in strange surroundings where housekeepers and maintenance people could freely come and go?

With some anxiety, I went on Amazon and ordered a steel security box, big enough for a laptop and some other things, like important papers. The box came, and it was massive. Heavy and awkward.

If this precious laptop had become my ego and my identity, and if I were to store this identity in this big steel box, my ego (and my anxiety) would become correspondingly massive. How depressing!

As it happened, the motel room had a security safe that sufficed. My massive lock box stayed in the trunk of the car. Was it my advancing age that made me anxious about the laptop? Was the contraction of our large house to a smallish motel room a stand-in for the inching proximity of illness and death? I don't know, but as we lugged our boxes and suitcases one by one up the stairs into this uncomfortable temporary abode, I felt small and vulnerable. And old. With each box, I felt my muscles and my tender back rebel. I felt not like myself—or the person I imagined myself to be. Or that I used to be.

The thought flitted into awareness and then just as quickly flitted out: I am old. I am too old for this. Isn't there someone out there who can help me?

Amy said the same thing, once all the boxes were safely inside our motel room. "I feel so old," she said. "I used to be able to cope with anything; I used to be able to do this without a problem. What happened to that younger person?" That's when we both realized that if we had waited even two or three years to engineer this huge move, we would have been too old to do it.

Others might wait longer. For us, we felt as if we had gotten out in the nick of time. No more forty stairs from the washer and dryer in the garage up to the second-story bedroom. No more lugging the trash bins down our steep driveway to the street. Whatever the future held, our aging bodies—especially my aging body—was free of those indignities. Forever.

Deep Mind Reflection: Home

I have spoken of our new house being our last house. I could also say *last home*, and when I do, I realize that the word *home* has a different tonality than *house.* My wife and I do once again have a home in a physical sense, and living here, we are home. But a home is not just a house. It is, in a psychic and emotional sense, who we really are, and the place within which we really live. That inner home is not any particular age. I'm not sure it really ages at all. Wherever we go, whatever we do, we are always home deep inside—though we may not always recognize it or acknowledge it.

Home has yet another meaning, one pertaining to the religious sphere. It is sometimes said that when a person dies, they are "going home." This has a particular meaning in Judeo-Christian belief, but regardless of your religious belief, dying as "going home" can simply mean that you are returning to the unknowable place you originally came from, when you were conceived or were born.

I also think that fully embracing our aging in all its aspects, its positives and negatives, with all the contradictory emotions that flourish within it, is still another kind of home. We could also call that embrace "coming home." Aging is coming home to who you really are—not who you used to be or who you imagine you still are, as a young man, vibrant and strong. Instead, come home to the reality of your aging body and aging mind, tending, in some respects, to waning and decline, but in others, growing into wisdom, mature judgment, and strength. This is the "holy grail" of the Parsifal legend of which Jungian author Robert E. Johnson speaks. We have been through many quests like Parsifal; we have suffered many wounds, we have won and lost innumerable battles, but, at last, our quest is done, and we can rest within the castle of our deepest home.

So for this final deep mind reflection, I suggest starting with the keyword *home.* I have already provided several different nuances of meaning of the word, but you should start fresh with your own blank slate. I think that when you intone the word, you will find that it has richness and depth. *Home, home*—the word is like the ringing of a bell. It sounds its initial strike, but the sound lingers for a long time.

Home. And as you repeat the striking of this bell, see what image comes to mind. Of course, you may first think of your home as the house you live in—the one where you may be sitting as you do this exercise. That is a physical space, but what of the emotional space that comes with it? How do you feel about being home? How do you feel when you walk through the door after a busy day, one day older than you were yesterday, and sit down in your favorite couch or chair? What is the feeling tone of that emotional home?

Tune in to the home that lives within your deep mind, that mind that itself is a kind of home, the place where all your memories, all your successes and failures, your nostalgia and regret, live and breathe. If you find that this is a place of comfort and safety, then you are living within the deep acceptance of which Erik Erikson speaks. Things may or may not have gone well in the full span of your life. Things may not be going well now. There may be trenchant worries and chronic concerns. But when you bring them home, when you embrace them from within your inner home, you can say to yourself, "I'm okay with all of this. I can go on."

The age you are, and the age you will be a year on or two years on, is part and parcel of your home. The people you love, and who love you, inhabit your home. The larger world has many problems. Maybe some of them keep you up at night, as they do me. Our town, our state, and our country are part of our home. The earth is our largest shared home. We are all aging in it and on it, every one of us—not just us human beings, but all living things.

Aging is what life does, and whatever happens tomorrow, next month, or next year, today we are all home together.

As your reflection into *home* comes to an end and dissipates into thin air, my wish for you is to continue aging well and to continue to grow and prosper into the time and place of your true, authentic home.

Endnotes

Chapter 1

1   Jim Ludes, "Of Bull Elephants and Mentors," Pell Center for International Relations and Public Policy, March 14, 2019, https://pellcenter.org/of-bull-elephants-and-mentors.

Chapter 3

1   "Will Sex Change as You Get Older?" Sexual Advice Association, April 19, 2016.

2   Irwin Goldstein, Amir Goren, Vicky W. Li, Martine C. Maculaitis, Wing Yu Tang, and Tarek A. Hassan, "The Association of Erectile Dysfunction with Productivity and Absenteeism in Eight Countries Globally," *International Journal of Clinical Practice* 73, no. 11 (2019): e13384.

3   Wikipedia, s.v. "Height discrimination," https://en.wikipedia.org/wiki/Height_discrimination.

Chapter 4

1   Gregory Warner, "How One Kenyan Tribe Produces the World's Best Runners," NPR, November 1, 2013, www.npr.org/sections/parallels/2013/11/01/241895965/how-one-kenyan-tribe-produces-the-worlds-best-runners.

2   Louann Brizandine, *The Female Brain* (New York: Broadway Books, 2006); Brizandine, *The Male Brain* (New York: Broadway Books, 2010). See also Audrey Nelson, "Why Don't Many Men Show Their Emotions?" *Psychology Today*, January 24, 2015, www.psychologytoday .com/us/blog/he-speaks-she-speaks/201501/why-don-t-many -men-show-their-emotions.

3   George F. Will, "Trump Doesn't Just Pollute the Social Environment with Hate. He Is the Environment," *Washington Post*, August 5, 2019.

4   Hilary Jacobs Hendel, "Emotions Are Physical," PsychCentral, July 8, 2018, https://psychcentral.com/blog/emotions-are-physical.

5   "Gender," *Psychology Today*, www.psychologytoday.com/us/basics /gender.

Chapter 5

1   Giuseppe Passarino, Francesco De ango, and Alberto Montesanto, "Human Longevity: Genetics or Lifestyle? It Takes Two to Tango," *Immunity and Ageing* 13 (2016), www.ncbi.nlm.nih.gov/pmc /articles/PMC4822264.

Chapter 6

1   "Marriage and Men's Health," Harvard Health Publishing, June 5, 2019, www.health.harvard.edu/mens-health/marriage-and -mens-health.

2   Rebecca Lee, "The Differences in Divorce for Men and Women," PsychCentral, July 8, 2018, https://psychcentral.com/blog/ the-differences-in-divorce-for-men-and-women.

Chapter 7

1   Michael Kinsley, "Mine Is Longer Than Yours," *New Yorker*, March 31, 2008, www.newyorker.com/magazine/2008/04/07/mine-is -longer-than-yours.

Chapter 8

1   Mandy Oaklander, "Old People Are Happier Than People in Their Twenties," *Time,* August 24, 2016, https://time.com/4464811/aging-happiness-stress-anxiety-depression.

2   Emily S. Rueb, "One in Ten Older Adults Binge Drinks, Study Says," New York Times, August 2, 2019, www.nytimes.com/2019/08/02/health/binge-drinkers-adult-alcohol.html.

3   Liz Mineo, "Good Genes Are Nice, but Joy Is Better," *The Harvard Gazette,* April 11, 2017, https://news.harvard.edu/gazette/story/2017/04/over-nearly-80-years-harvard-study-has-been-showing-how-to-live-a-healthy-and-happy-life.

Chapter 9

1   Barbara A. Friedberg, "Are We in a Baby Boomer Retirement Crisis?" Investopedia, September 23, 2019, www.investopedia.com/articles/personal-finance/032216/are-we-baby-boomer-retirement-crisis.asp.

2   Andrew Soergel, "Poll: 1 in 4 Don't Plan to Retire Despite Realities of Aging," KCBE, July 7, 2019, www.kcbd.com/2019/07/07/poll-dont-plan-retire-despite-realities-aging.

3   Pat Eaton-Robb, "Lawyer, 99, Will Retire 'When They Carry Me Out of Here.'" *Fox News,* September 30, 2018, www.foxnews.com/us/lawyer-99-will-retire-when-they-carry-me-out-of-here.

Chapter 10

1   "Oxytocin for Women," Oxytocin Accelerator, www.oxytocinaccelerator.com/oxytocin-and-women.

Index

About the Author

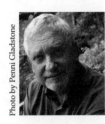

Photo by Penni Gladstone

LEWIS RICHMOND has been a meditation teacher, musician, and software entrepreneur. He is the author of four previous books, including the national best-seller, *Work as a Spiritual Practice: A Practical Buddhist Approach to Inner Growth and Satisfaction on the Job* and the more recent award-winning *Aging as a Spiritual Practice: A Contemplative Guide to Growing Older and Wiser*. In addition to these books, Richmond's essays have appeared in such magazines as *Tricycle*, *The Buddhadharma*, *Turning Wheel*, and *Shambhala Sun*. While in retirement, he remains a musician and composer, and an editor and mentor to other authors.

To connect with Lewis Richmond, go to www.LewisRichmond.com.

About North Atlantic Books

North Atlantic Books (NAB) is an independent, nonprofit publisher committed to a bold exploration of the relationships between mind, body, spirit, and nature. Founded in 1974, NAB aims to nurture a holistic view of the arts, sciences, humanities, and healing. To make a donation or to learn more about our books, authors, events, and newsletter, please visit www.northatlanticbooks.com.

North Atlantic Books is the publishing arm of the Society for the Study of Native Arts and Sciences, a 501(c)(3) nonprofit educational organization that promotes cross-cultural perspectives linking scientific, social, and artistic fields. To learn how you can support us, please visit our website.